THE
SOUL
MIDWIVES'
HANDBOOK

First published and distributed in the United Kingdom by:
Hay House UK Ltd, Astley House, 33 Notting Hill Gate, London W11 3JQ
Tel: +44 (0)20 3675 2450; Fax: +44 (0)20 3675 2451
www.hayhouse.co.uk

Published and distributed in the United States of America by:
Hay House Inc., PO Box 5100, Carlsbad, CA 92018-5100
Tel: (1) 760 431 7695 or (800) 654 5126
Fax: (1) 760 431 6948 or (800) 650 5115
www.hayhouse.com

Published and distributed in Australia by:
Hay House Australia Ltd, 18/36 Ralph St, Alexandria NSW 2015
Tel: (61) 2 9669 4299; Fax: (61) 2 9669 4144
www.hayhouse.com.au

Published and distributed in the Republic of South Africa by:
Hay House SA (Pty) Ltd, PO Box 990, Witkoppen 2068
Tel/Fax: (27) 11 467 8904
www.hayhouse.co.za

Published and distributed in India by:
Hay House Publishers India, Muskaan Complex, Plot No.3, B-2,
Vasant Kunj, New Delhi 110 070
Tel: (91) 11 4176 1620; Fax: (91) 11 4176 1630
www.hayhouse.co.in

Distributed in Canada by:
Raincoast, 9050 Shaughnessy St, Vancouver BC V6P 6E5
Tel: (1) 604 323 7100; Fax: (1) 604 323 2600

A catalogue record for this book is available from the British Library.

ISBN: 978-1-84850-703-6

Printed and bound by TJ International Ltd, Padstow, Cornwall

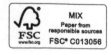

MIX
Paper from
responsible sources
FSC® C013056

Praise for *The Soul Midwives' Handbook*:

'In this moving book, Felicity has encapsulated the wisdom of the ages into practical examples of how to BE with the dying; how to honour and hold that sacred space for everyone as they prepare to make the journey that we all must take.'
Anita Moorjani, author of *Dying to Be Me*

'It is wonderful that Felicity Warner's Soul Midwives now have a handbook for practical use. As vigiling reclaims its rightful place at the bedside, The Soul Midwives' Handbook *emerges as a useful and timely tool for those who are called to this sacred work.'*
Megory Anderson PhD, author of *Sacred Dying*

'Well, don't they do fantastic work?
Not just for the dying, but for those left behind.'
Brian Blessed, actor

'The work of Felicity Warner and the Soul Midwives is absolutely crucial for those of us who believe that death is one of the most important moments of our life. By providing loving and gentle support, Felicity and the Soul Midwives support people to have the death that they want. What could be more important?'
Jon Underwood, pioneer of the Death Cafe movement

Praise for *A Safe Journey Home*, also by Felicity Warner:

*'Soul midwives make it their mission to help the dying
pass away with dignity and in peace.'*
Sunday Express

'The woman who wants to make dying more dignified.'
Woman's Weekly

*'A guide to help people prepare for death just as they might for a birth –
and achieve a peaceful end to their lives.'*
You magazine

'A gift for bringing comfort and peace to those who are about to pass away.'
Daily Express

*'Offers guidance and practical advice on how to offer support
and care to those on the final journey.'*
Yoga and Health magazine

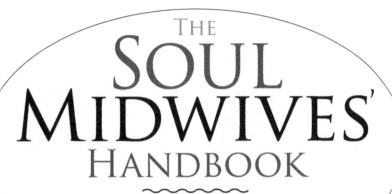

THE SOUL MIDWIVES' HANDBOOK

The Holistic & Spiritual Care of the Dying

FELICITY WARNER

Founder of the Soul Midwives' Movement

HAY HOUSE

Carlsbad, California • New York City • London • Sydney
Johannesburg • Vancouver • Hong Kong • New Delhi

❧ CONTENTS ❧

❧ PREFACE ❧

Just as I began to write this book I heard the sad news that Gill Edwards, my dear and treasured friend, had died.

Gill was well known for her books on spirituality and energy medicine and was one of the most inspiring teachers of our time. For me, she was also something of a spiritual godmother and probably the first person to encourage me to use my gifts as a healer and seer.

We met many years ago, just as her first book, *Living Magically*, was published. We sat in her sunny cottage, eating lunch and exploring ideas for an article I'd been commissioned to write about her transition from NHS psychologist to spiritual writer. We instantly realized we had a deep connection and lost no time in talking about everything from angels to shamanism, healing, vibrational medicine, psychology and soul retrieval, the invisible realms and a vast world of things I'd never even heard of.

As dusk fell, and with gallons of tea consumed, I remember feeling completely intoxicated with joy and inspiration.

Just before I left, I asked Gill for one final nugget of advice for anyone questing for a spiritual life.

'Tell them they should all "follow their bliss",' she laughed. 'That's the real key to living magically.'

I gathered my notebooks and pens and Gill helped me carry my things to the car before asking, very seriously, 'What's *your* bliss, Felicity? When are you going to begin *your* real work and start to use the magic that you've been blessed with? You have a long trail of ancestors stretching behind you waiting for you to begin your soul work. It's time to honour them and use the gifts they have given you. Don't take too long to follow your bliss. None of us is here for long.'

I left feeling puzzled but curious. I knew she'd spoken the truth, but it still took me a few years to get there. Eventually, however, my work in honouring the ancestors became my service in creating Soul Midwifery. Thanks, Gill, for the nudge!

Gill understood the deeper mysteries of life and death and knew how to explain them with simplicity and honesty. She saw the truth, beauty and spirit in everything around her. Her teaching was always engaging, direct and bold. Her graceful death in November 2011 inspired so many people. Her family has agreed to let me share her final letter to her friends, explaining how she felt as she stepped across the sacred threshold:

> *I'm so sorry that some of you may be feeling grief and loss. I think the loss of someone we love is perhaps the hardest challenge that anyone ever has to face, so my heart goes out to you. What I can say is that we can make the experience far worse, or far better, by the way we see it. As I understand it, pain always means that we are not seeing things as our higher self sees them (which is why we feel negative emotion – as a warning sign of this splitting of energy).*
>
> *If you have been touched by my death then my understanding is that you and I had a contract to part around this time, for all the gifts that it would eventually bring to you – which you will only understand when you look back in years to come. You may have done some workshops with me, and I'm sure you know (in theory) that*

death is not a tragedy; it is simply the choice to make a transition from one state of consciousness to another. Yes, it would be easier if I had chosen just to retire and no longer respond to emails, but somehow you have to come to terms with the choice I made. For whatever reasons, this lifetime was finished for me.

I am still very much here, just not embodied any more. Love is an eternal bond, and you only need to think of me with love and I will be there, connecting with you. But you will only be able to sense me when you release the grief and simply connect with the love. (A friend of mine even co-authored a book with a close friend after her friend's death, having established close and easy communication with her.) You might be amazed at how rapidly you can find peace again, once you get your energy flowing and reconnect with your higher self (who sees nothing as bad or wrong).

You can focus on what is wrong or missing – my death – or you can choose to focus on what is positive. I have gone physically but I am absolutely fine, and you are still here – and so many good times lie in store for you still, with many other people to love and be loved by. If you look for what is positive in life, and things to be grateful for in each day, and choose to think only of happy memories of me, you will begin to release the grief – and then you will begin to attract more positive events and opportunities into your life. Focus on what you enjoy, whom you enjoy being with and what dreams you have for the future. It might take time, but you can do it. In the meantime, there are hundreds of comforting books about the afterlife which show beyond any doubt that life is eternal, and that the only reality is Love.

I wish you all the very best with your journey. It will get easier – and so many gifts lie ahead.

With love and blessings,

Gill

Gill was a guiding light and teacher and respected friend, and I thank her for encouraging me to begin my own journey and to follow the unexpected pathway that has led to creating the craft of Soul Midwifery

❧ ACKNOWLEDGEMENTS ❧

This book has taken many years to grow, and so there are many people I would like to thank.

I am very grateful to the family of Gill Edwards for agreeing to let me share Gill's final letter to her friends.

Thank you also to:

Michelle Pilley and her wonderful team at Hay House for their constant encouragement and support.

Chelsey Fox of Fox & Howard Literary Agency.

Mandy Preece, tutor at the Soul Midwives' School, for her goodness, fun, bright eyes and magic wand.

Michael Chamberlain, Dee Dade and Elizabeth Hornby for being wise, inspiring and humorous tutors at the Soul Midwives' School, and to Elizabeth for her prayers and healing music.

Antonia Rolls, Ann Freeman, Gail Dyson, Helen Fields, Theo Hall and Susan Palumbo for allowing me to share their stories.

Mike Dooley for agreeing to me using his 10 things the dying wish to tell us.

Anita Moorjani for permission to use an extract from her book *Dying to Be Me*.

Christine Longaker for use of her exercise in how dying feels.

The artist Dan Chen for agreeing to let me describe his end-of-life hospital project.

Charlotte Gush for her blessing.

All the families and 'friends' with whom I have worked over many years. You have 'woven a cloak around my heart'.

The team of teachers who have 'midwived' my soul and continue to teach me, with boundless patience, the inner and outer mysteries of transition and consciousness.

And last but not least, my own wonderful family:

Richard, who keeps the hearth glowing with sturdy logs and bright sparks to welcome all the hundreds of people into our sanctuary and home.

My two beautiful daughters, Daisy and Lusea, who thrived and blossomed despite having a quirky mother who believed in moss-poultices rather than plasters.

My parents, Noëlle and David, for both daring to be different, and my darling granddaughters, Matilda and Amelie, who are the joy of life itself.

∾ INTRODUCTION ∾

A middle-aged woman is curled up in a foetal position on a mattress on the floor. She doesn't look up and is clearly very close to death. One of her skeletal arms is wired up to an electronic device which is plugged in beside her.

A doctor in a pristine white coat crouches down to check her vital signs before signing a form confirming that death is imminent.

Checking that there's no more to be done, he quietly fiddles with some knobs and dials and sets the machines. A panel of lights comes on with a hiss of whirring dials. Without looking at the woman again, the doctor sets the volume control and leaves the room, shutting the door quietly behind him.

The LED lights up and displays the words 'Detecting end of life'.

A second later, the machine switches on and a robotic arm begins to stroke the dying woman's arm. Back and forth it caresses her and then an automated voice message starts:

I am the Last Moment Robot. I am here to help you and guide you
through your last moment on Earth. I am sorry that your family and
friends can't be with you right now, but don't be afraid. I am here
to comfort you. You are not alone, you are with me. Your family and
friends love you very much; they will remember you after you are gone.

Is this a chilling glimpse of palliative care in the near future?

Luckily not! It is an art installation called 'Last Moment Hospital' created by Dan Chen, an American artist, designer and engineer. It's designed to shock; it hits you in the heart and makes you think deeply about intimacy and how we care for the dying.

The robot strokes the dying woman, trying to comfort her while its staccato electronic voice personalizes the recorded message with her name.

Dan Chen explains that his installation reveals the cruelty of life and the lack of human support and social connections that some people experience:

> ...it also makes viewers think about the placebo effects of comfort... Is it better to have a robot talking to you as you die, or nothing at all? Ultimately, what is intimacy without humanity?

Approximately 100,000 people die every day, but how many of us have thought about how we would like to die? In the West, death happens mostly in hospitals, care homes or hospices. And, sadly, most of us are terrified by the thought of it.

The majority of people simply choose not to think about death until it literally stares them in the face. According to the UK organization Dying Matters, 81 per cent of people in Britain have not written down any preferences around their own death, and only a quarter of men and just over one in three women have told anyone about the funeral arrangements they would like to have. Nearly two-thirds of people have not written a will, including a quarter of the over-65s.

Moreover, every year a fifth of NHS beds are taken up with end-of-life care, yet two out of five people who die in hospital have conditions that medicine cannot help. And 60 per cent of NHS complaints concern end-of-life care.

What of those who have considered their own death? According to a YouGov poll, two out of three people would prefer to die at home, and 90 per cent of those dying in hospital would rather die at home. Yet half of us will die in a care home or hospital.

Happily, the tide is slowly turning. Many more people are talking openly about death, thinking about their own mortality and exploring the options facing them – determining to make it a better experience not just for themselves but also for the loved ones left behind. More people are requesting to die at home, with their families around them, just as people did in times past. Soul Midwives are there to ease this journey.

A Soul Midwife is the very opposite of a dying-room robot. Our bedside care is tender, personal and very human. Instead of robots for the dying, we will find Soul Midwives in every hospice, hospital and care home within the next few years. Already you'll find them in many care settings, as well as working with people dying at home. Although Soul Midwives have esoteric knowledge of certain aspects of dying, they are also practical and down-to-earth and work alongside medical teams. There are Soul Midwives who specialize in working with children, with people with learning disabilities, those with Alzheimer's or other mental health problems, or in just about every situation you can imagine.

There have, of course, always been people who have sat with the dying. Traditionally, Soul Midwifery (although it didn't have the name then) was a sacred service passed to adepts by their masters through outer and inner teachings based on an oral tradition. The techniques were practised by only the very highest initiates once they had proved their dedication to others and their self-mastery. This handbook draws on these ancient traditions and shares the outer teachings, with small references to the deeper levels of the work.

My own quest for knowledge has led me to wise elders, holy men and women, nuns, priests, musicians, healers, artists and celebrants. I have scoured every religion, from Buddhism to Islam, Paganism and various forms of Christianity, absorbing the wisdom of their traditions. I believe that many of the rituals and holistic practices observed for thousands of years by indigenous groups to nurture and soothe the dying hold clues to helping us all to die well.

Above all, however, being a Soul Midwife is based on deep soul friendship. This is why I have given the name 'friend' to the people we serve.

I have sought the permission of the friends whose stories I tell here, except where so much detail has been changed that the subject cannot be identified. The intimacy of these stories contains a profound quality of truth which has proved time and again to me that death isn't the end, just the closing of one chapter of the soul and the beginning of a new one.

This book is also the story of my own journey in unscrambling the lost knowledge of Soul Midwifery and fine-tuning it to provide a practical resource for today's modern healthcare.

My work began over 20 years ago. At the time I was a health journalist covering hard-nosed clinical and surgical procedures in hi-tech hospital medicine. I was writing a series of in-depth articles about what it was like to die young. Several young women in the final stages of breast cancer offered to tell me how it was for them. Over time, as their health deteriorated, I got to know them all on a very deep level. Their experiences, which I describe in detail in my previous book, *A Safe Journey Home*, amazed and also saddened me. Their understanding of death and dying shone a light on their hopes and fears, but also on other people's reactions and projections. From them I learned the practical difficulties of being ill and also the extreme spiritual challenges.

Although none of these women would have termed themselves spiritual in any way, each experienced a complex existential unfolding which brought with it profound spiritual insights. I watched them all adapt and grow into a deeper aspect of themselves. They became truly wise women, speaking their truth in a very liberated way as they journeyed out of life.

Working with these sharp, sassy, fearless women was an exciting time. I had no experience of offering spiritual companionship as such, but it seemed to develop as we swam together, exploring new territory which was characterized by deeply soulful exchanges. They told me how it really felt to be dying, and what they were experiencing underneath the surface. They wanted their deaths to be significant and inspiring. And they were – these women were the trendsetters for a new way of thinking.

After sharing their experiences and all the miraculous – and harrowing – events that came with them, I felt as if I had come home to myself and was involved in work that I had somehow done before. I began volunteering at a local hospice and sitting with others close to death.

It is now many years since I began working with the dying, but I'll never forget the first time that I held a young woman's hand as she slipped away. She'd been restless and terrified, and had no family or friends to comfort her. I had been asked to sit with her, as she was agitated and constantly crying out. All I could think was, *What would her mother do if she was here?* So I found her hand and told her that I would stay with her. She stopped crying and turned and looked at me, and I began to sing.

A warm cloak pulled in around us and I could feel her fear begin to ebb away. She knew she was dying and that there was no turning back, but her body – and soul – knew what to do. Feeling safe with someone holding her hand, she surrendered and grew calmer. Despite the pain and anxiety, there was also a feeling that all was well. And it was. She died very peacefully a few hours later.

Her death, an initiation for both of us, showed me how miraculous and rich a good death could be.

Gradually I began to see a pattern in the deaths around me. There were definite stages covering physical, emotional and spiritual shifts. I could see that on a very primal level there was a common experience of dying that was somehow being missed or overlooked in the busy medical context. I became curious to learn more.

One day, sitting and feeling rather spare and useless, I had a lightbulb moment and intuited (perhaps romantically) that there must once have been a body of knowledge, or an archaic system, that was the key to supporting, at a soul level, someone who was dying.

Suddenly, things began to fall into place. The clues were everywhere: in traditional and indigenous societies, in the great Eastern religions, in medical traditions... There were many different practices – both simple and complicated – to respect the act of dying as a sacred time.

I began writing about my experiences and talking to anyone who would listen, and then people started finding me – doctors, priests, nurses, social workers, therapists and, most importantly, ordinary people with no special skills other than experience of life.

I learned some important lessons that totally altered my understanding of death. I realized that:

- Death is an illusion. The body dies, but the soul does not.

- There is survival of consciousness.

- Death is a process involving mind, body and soul.

- A good death is a wonder. It is a healing experience for everyone involved – something to be celebrated.

- Dying is a process of shedding and releasing: each shift enables a different set of experiences to be resolved.

- We expect pain, fear and sadness amongst the dying, but there can also be a strong sense of the soul blossoming, a quickening and transformation and a divine sense of grace.

- There is a divine grace and rhythm to the whole dying process.

- When we make friends with death we are shown how to truly live.

Somehow, strangely, modern Western medicine had no view of this.

Gradually, I became more confident at the bedside – sometimes offering gentle hand massage or simple healing, sometimes playing soothing music, but mainly just listening and being fully present.

After a few visits, the dying person often appeared to cheer up and feel a bit better. Was it that the atmosphere around them had changed? At that time I didn't know much about energy medicine, but companionship, listening, holding hands and a little bit of singing seemed to work wonders. Something seemed to shift and the gloom would lift.

These interludes were brief, like bursts of sunshine in winter, but they raised the spirits and often gave my dying friends enough energy to see visitors or make important phone calls. I received many texts asking for 'top-ups', as my friends felt stronger and lighter after a visit.

But always, as death approached, their focus would shift from wanting to keep going as normal to needing a cocoon so that they could focus on their inner worlds. As time passed, they would enter a different, more serene space.

I made these visits in my spare time, often feeling quite overwhelmed afterwards by the intensity of the experience and the privilege of being able to help. And I wasn't only helping the dying person – families, as I gradually got to know them, would ask me to be there to support them as well.

One day someone called me at home and asked to speak to the 'Soul Midwife'. It was the first time my work had been given a name, and somehow it stuck.

I have now trained many Soul Midwives, both women and men, who have taken the work far and wide in Europe, America, New Zealand, Australia and Canada, working in hospices and care homes and people's homes and at the heart of the community. These very special practitioners are devoted to easing the pain of others. They have extended my original vision, transforming it into something larger and braver than I would ever have dared to envisage by myself.

If you would like to be part of this new way of working with the dying, this handbook will guide you. In opening up your heart to the care of the dying you will be making a powerful change, not only to your own life but also to the lives of those for whom you care. Your journey will be incredible – hard at times, but always imbued with a sense of the miraculous.

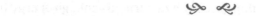

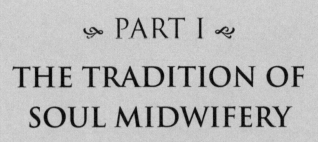

✎ PART I ✎

THE TRADITION OF SOUL MIDWIFERY

'Death is but a doorway to a new life.
We live today. We shall live again.
In many forms we shall return to this Earth.'

Ancient Egyptian proverb

CHAPTER 1

ANCIENT SECRETS AND SACRED RITES

'Gently, gently... breathing, softly, in,
gently, gently... "You are doing so well," she whispers, "so, so well."
She sings to me... a tune my mother sang...
I am wrapped, held safe with her love.
She leads me to the sea of my heart.
The boat is waiting.
We sail together... to the far horizon.
"What can you see?" she asks.
"What can you see?"
Then she takes my hand
and I fall asleep.'

FELICITY WARNER

Although the title 'Soul Midwife' is modern, the role we offer is as ancient as humankind. As a tribe, we have always known how to sit with the dying and soften the final hours. It has always been the work of Soul

Midwives to ease the pain, to soothe the wound, to calm the breath, to feel the pulse, to keep the soul warm, to feed the hearth with sticks and logs. To sing the songs that ask the ancestors to guide the spirit of the dying one home. To pray and bless and wash the body, close the eyes, blend the oils, mix the herbs, stew the tea, calm the dog, protect the loved ones. To honour and release the bones, and wrap them in binding cloths to sleep in the soft dark earth. It is only in the last 60 years or so that we have lost touch with these skills, as dying people have been taken away to die in hospitals, hospices and care homes rather than in their own beds or in the heart of the home by the warming fire.

The art of dying well used to be taught widely. It was regarded as an important life skill in many civilizations – Egypt, Tibet, India and throughout Europe into the Middle Ages. The instructions, or *ars moriendi* (the art of dying), consisted of prayers and reflections, spiritual practices and in some traditions bodywork such as yoga and specific breathing techniques, and were designed to guide initiates through their dying in the hope of peaceful refuge in the afterlife. Many of my ideas and inspirations have been collected and adapted from a variety of sources that draw on these ancient traditions, including indigenous communities, folk medicine, shamanic practice and the inner mystery traditions of several of the world's great religions.

There are countless stories of early Soul Midwifery. In ancient Hebrew, Sumerian and Egyptian times, priestesses were trained in music, healing arts and high magic, using chant, sacred dance and healing herbs. These wise women carried great wisdom and knowledge, which was often viewed as a threat. During the fourth century AD, the Roman Emperor Constantine and the Council of Nicea eventually decreed that women would be banned from speaking or singing in church, and gradually the healing traditions of women across the Mediterranean and Europe were forced underground.

Only scattered remnants of these traditions are left today, as very little was written down. The inner secrets of transition were carefully guarded, as knowledge without wisdom can be dangerous. Yet clues to the mysteries are all around us.

According to the ancient Sanskrit text the *Bhagavad Gita*, the great secret of the universe is contained within three mysteries of death and the soul:

- The first mystery is to be found in human consciousness. It is something we already know in our bones and in our collective memory. The path to remembering has to be intuited, however, and can arise only when an individual has begun deep inner questioning. This knowingness ripens on the inner planes and is not dependent on any outside teaching or being revealed by a master.

- The second mystery is that practising in accordance with the secret and its wisdom has to be righteous, morally lawful and in accordance with the rules of the cosmos and universal principles.

- Thirdly, it must be 'pleasant beyond measure'. The secret and its wisdom must be life-enhancing, and above the pleasures and limits of earthly existence.

These teachings still apply today and are still carefully guarded. It takes years to work at such a deep level. The inner teachings are still passed between master and pupil in stages, and only after the pupil has successfully passed through a strict series of tests, rituals and initiation ceremonies. The esoteric aspects of Soul Midwifery continue to be 'hidden in plain sight', only appearing to those who have eyes to see and ears to hear. Many of them are preserved in code amongst other archaic information.

The esoteric aspects of Soul Midwifery don't appeal to everyone, of course, and it isn't essential to practise them in order to help the dying. If you feel that you would like to work on a very simple level, such as holding hands and keeping someone company, that is good Soul Midwifery too.

Today more and more Soul Midwives are encompassing the work of the old priestesses and wise women and reintroducing the sacred to the care of the dying within mainstream healthcare. See what captures your imagination after reading the descriptions below. Once you start uncovering the treasures that line the path before you, your work will be forever enriched by them.

TRADITIONS

Throughout the oldest myths and folk stories we find rich pockets of wisdom on helping the dying to pass gently from this life to the next. The ancient world also gives us many valuable traditions. The Egyptians, Babylonians, Chinese, Tibetans and indigenous peoples of South America all believed that the soul survived death and gave instructions on reaching the afterlife.

The Egyptians

The Egyptians also had a sophisticated concept of the cosmology of the soul. They believed that humans consisted of the physical body (the Ka) and the personality or spirit (the Ba) and that the heart was the chief centre of consciousness. This thinking is very in tune with the view of Soul Midwives today and with our own understanding regarding the physical body and the lightbody (the subtle energetic bodies, or energetic signature, of a person).

A collection of the Egyptians' teachings – the Egyptian *Book of the Dead*, also known as the chapter of *Coming Forth by Day* – formed a guide to death and the afterlife, and consisted of incantations, spells and precise formulae to guide the dead to the underworld.

What the Egyptians taught Soul Midwives:

- the power of myth
- the use of symbols (for anointing, and as energy symbols such as those we see in modern Reiki)
- the use of anointing oils
- energy techniques
- initiations for mastery of the physical body.

The Hathors

Hathor was an Egyptian goddess. One of her titles was Mistress of the West and her responsibilities included welcoming the dead into the next life. She was a goddess of music and sound, as well as being a spiritual midwife protecting women giving birth. Many temples were dedicated to her, but the most important was at Dendera. It is believed that her temple priestesses, the Hathors, entered trance states (perhaps induced by snake bites) to channel her teachings.

Hathor is interesting to Soul Midwives because her teachings explain how to work with the soul by using sound. Perhaps this is the origin of toning – creating single-syllable sounds with the voice – as one of the Hathors' teachings says that our voices are healing tools. By toning, we can create powerful healing fields around the dying.

The Hathors are also thought to have shown how we can move energy through the body in a spiralling motion, releasing emotions, memories and soul wounds (*see pages 75–76*) and rebalancing the energy field.

What the Hathors taught Soul Midwives:

- how to work with sound, vibration and resonance

- how to spin the energy field

- the power of the human voice.

Myrrhophores

The myrrhophores, or myrrh bearers, were priestesses of transition and advanced soul technicians. They may have originated from the Egyptian temples of the goddess Isis, but their work is more widely known through the Bible, especially the crucifixion. The most famous myrrhophore is Mary Magdalene.

As well as preparing people for death, the myrrhophores healed physical conditions by placing oils on their fingertips and then spinning them through the chakras, or energy centres, of the body, in a process mentioned in the Egyptian *Book of the Dead* as 'Cleansing of the Flesh and Blood'.

Their outer, visible work was to prepare the body prior to burial, but in their inner work they used many high-frequency oils such as spikenard, frankincense, myrrh and cedar for transition and after-death support. They understood that high-frequency oils magnified the lightbody, and they were able to raise or lower a person's vibration. They could also manifest energy as pure colour.

Their knowledge disappeared underground for many centuries, but it's now reappearing. A very small number of people are the wisdom-keepers for their craft.

What the myrrhophores taught Soul Midwives:

- the esoteric science of working with oils and energy to prepare people for transition

- how to work with the lightbody and the soul

- how to work with colour and crystalline energy.

The Essenes

The Essenes were a Jewish sect known for their prophetic, devotional, spiritual and healing work. Jesus is thought to have lived in an Essene community during his early life and to have studied their healing methods.

The word 'Essene' means 'healer' or 'therapeutic', and the Essenes were masters of energy medicine. Their teachings and philosophy on how to live were influenced by Brahmanism, the ancient Hindu texts of the Vedas and the Upanishads, and the yoga systems of India.

Schooled in philosophy and metaphysics, the Essenes had a very 'green' outlook on life. They did not eat meat and lived gently and peacefully in small communities away from towns and villages. They studied the weather and knew how the elements and seasons affected the nutrients in the soil. Food was grown not only to nourish but also to heal. The Essenes also fasted regularly and knew how to rejuvenate and restore their bodies by working with their energy fields.

Washing the feet, hands and body was very important, and the Essenes physically and spiritually cleansed themselves each morning and evening, and before eating, praying or working. One of their customs was to wash the feet of their friends and neighbours as a sign of devotion and humility, and to show that they cared deeply for everyone around them.

They also blessed each other by laying their hands on the top of the head. This gesture was thought to bring healing light down and ensure that everyone was a clear channel for the light. Perhaps it was also a technique of chakra balancing.

The Essenes also knew how to use their voices to cure illness and to prepare people for death.

What the Essenes taught Soul Midwives:

- how to work with love, respect and humility

- how to create compassionate communities

9

- how to heal with hands and voices

- advanced healing methods

- the importance of diet, cleanliness and spiritual practice for physical and spiritual wellbeing.

Tibetan Buddhists

The most useful diagnostic practices guiding Soul Midwives stem from Eastern medicine, particularly Chinese and Tibetan. These energy-based approaches might seem whacky to Western minds, but they are grounded in scientific fact.

The Chinese and Tibetan systems are based on the view that human bodies are instruments of energy. How we breathe, the colour and coating of our tongue and the quality and character of our internal pulse all give important clues to the *chi*, or life force, we contain. These pointers, the basics of modern energy medicine, begin to make perfect sense when we see them in the context of the human energy field.

Like the Egyptians, the Tibetans had their 'books of the dead': a collection of texts which were not only guidebooks for the deceased but also important spiritual writings.

The Tibetans developed an exact science out of the process of dying and the survival of consciousness, and Buddhist teachers throughout the centuries have guided their students in meditation on death and impermanence. The Tibetan understanding of the dying process has become the foundation of the Soul Midwives' diagnostic model.

Central to the Tibetan concept of afterlife existence is the Bardo, which literally means 'intermediate state'. There is in fact a sequence of states or stages (Bardos) through which the individual passes between death and rebirth.

Like many other traditions, the Tibetan recognizes that subtle consciousness may remain in the body for about three days after death. Tibetans believe that the body should be left undisturbed during that time, as any disruption may affect the transfer of consciousness. For 49 days after death, prayers will be said for the soul to take it through the Bardo state.

What the Tibetan Buddhists taught Soul Midwives:

• the meaning of life/impermanence/suffering

• the cosmology of the soul

• the states of consciousness after death.

The Shamanic Traditions

Shamans (traditional healers and medicine men or women) enter other states of consciousness to communicate with animals, elements of nature and beings from other realms. When they journey with the dying, they may meet spirit guides, power animals and ancestors relating to the person concerned and retrieve information and guidance.

All shamanic traditions celebrate rituals around dying, but these vary between communities. One of the rituals, called the *Despacho*, centres around burning a prayer bundle made from paper, fabric or even pieces of old clothing, which represents the dying person's life. As the bundle burns, the soul is transformed and cleansed for the next part of its journey.

Another very important part of the shaman's work which relates to Soul Midwifery is soul retrieval. Here the shaman journeys on behalf of the friend to retrieve soul parts which have been lost due to trauma during life. Restoring these parts to make the soul whole again before transition can help a person to die well.

What the shamanic traditions taught Soul Midwives:

- how to support and make whole the soul of a friend
- how to work with people who are unconscious in the form of merging and journeying
- how to call in the ancestors to assist with transition.

Celtic Traditions

The Celtic way of Soul Midwifery is to assist transition by creating an atmosphere of beauty and tenderness through poetry, music and ritual. The wise women in Ireland, Scotland, Wales and Cornwall not only sat and watched over the dying, but also healed the community by singing laments and 'keening' for the dead one.

Lamenting was a tradition to honour the dead and also to help the mourners openly express and release their sorrow. As well as singing, the women would utter loud piercing wails, sometimes accompanied by music.

Traditional Irish wakes involve all-night vigils around the corpse before the funeral, with poetry and storytelling. The Irish consider keening to be part of a spiritual language which is heard by the dead as they journey.

Green medicine, using herbs and tree essences, etc., is also part of the Celtic traditions.

What the Celtic traditions taught Soul Midwives:

- vigiling
- the importance of working with beauty and the soul
- music
- poetry
- laments

- keening

- herbal medicine

- myths

Curanderismo

Curanderismo is a form of folk medicine practised mainly in South America. It is a mixture of many traditions, including gypsy, Spanish/ Moorish, shamanic and Mayan. It uses many techniques for healing, including herbalism, massage and rituals for dealing with curses and spirit possession.

Curanderos try to show how the person manifested their illness in the first place. They act as mirrors, revealing what needs to be healed on a personal and spiritual level. Working with heart energy and a link to source, they also honour our connection to Mother Earth.

Many natural tools are used in their healing practices, such as stones, wood, crystals and feathers. Herbs are also used to make healing teas.

What *curanderos* taught Soul Midwives:

- that the divine is the healing force, not us

- the importance of treating the whole person – mind, body and soul

- the recognition that physical illness has its root in soul 'dis-ease'

- that most diseases occur as a result of other people's connection to us

- the value of combining healing with massage and ritual

- the importance of storytelling

- how to work with the help of our ancestors.

The ancestors from the various traditions mentioned above are still present, weaving their teachings into our modern practices. They have walked this far and now we must walk the rest of the way.

THE SOUL MIDWIVES' LINEAGE

We lost a tender part of our group soul when we forgot how to sit with the dying; when we forgot the value of holding hands and placing our loved ones beside the glowing embers of their own hearths; when we decided that machinery was more important, and that a germ-free environment with easy-to-clean surfaces was a better place in which to die.

Imagine the exquisite connection that the Inuit feel when gazing into the night sky and seeing the dancing northern lights, the *aurora borealis*, as torches that guide souls towards heaven. Imagine seeing, in the shadows, the myrrhophores, the myrrh-bearing women who tend the dying with aromatic oils, or the ancestors who come to lead the way home. Remember the traditional wise women and men who lived in the homesteads, the villages, out in the forests, beside the rivers, up steep wooded mountains, in towns and communities everywhere humanity has ever lived, sitting with the dying, soothing and healing with herbs and music, vigiling, singing the soul home, preparing the body for the wake...

This is where you'll find the lineage of Soul Midwives, weaving their way through time; men and women who silently but diligently held the space for the dying and created the sacred passings for generations of souls throughout history.

Archetypes within the planet's myths and legends also reveal a history of supporting mind, body and soul.

An affinity to a specific historical or archetypal Soul Midwife may reveal a particular skill or way that you may choose to work. Here are some examples:

Mary Magdalene

Mary Magdalene is said by some to have been the first ever Soul Midwife, holding the energy when Christ died on the cross. She was a teacher and lineage-holder of the great Egyptian mystery teachings of Isis. She used profound energy techniques to assist transition at a deep soul level.

Healer Soul Midwives are attracted to her strong teachings, which are still being revealed.

Angels

Angels are seen as carers of the soul in many of the world's major traditions. They are considered to be protectors of the sick and vulnerable, personal guides and always in loving service of humanity and at hand to sit with the dying and their families. Many salt-of-the-earth Soul Midwives are guided and taught by angels.

Brigit

Brigit is the renowned Celtic Soul Midwife. As well as being a silversmith, poet and blacksmith, she teaches the esoteric secrets of her craft from her cauldron of wisdom. She has an alliance with other beings, such as fairies and elementals, and soothes the dying with a mixture of poetry, music and singing.

Music therapists and creative Soul Midwives resonate strongly with her teachings.

Healer/Teacher Figures

Florence Nightingale, Elizabeth Fry, Dame Cicely Saunders and Mother Teresa of Calcutta all used their charisma and skills to improve the journey of the dying. They all lived in a way that inspired others and taught by example.

If you are drawn to these figures, this might indicate a path of using Soul Midwifery skills in a practical, therapeutic or medical context.

Hecate

Hecate is possibly the most challenging of the archetypes. As goddess of the crossroads, with the power to see past, present and future, she has the gift of clairvoyant sight and the ability to see the soul. Her wisdom interprets knowledge and prevents us from working with our intellect. She demands we see the bigger picture and think from the heart. She is tough, challenging and always brings attention to the shadow side in order to balance it with the light. She has the power to take us into difficult places, such as prisons, to do our work with those who have had difficult lives, for example people suffering from addiction.

Holy Men and Women

Jesus, the Buddha and St Francis of Assisi are all iconic figures of selfless service to the dying, impoverished and unloved. They inspire us to work amongst the poor, the lonely and the disadvantaged, especially abroad or amongst impoverished communities.

If you are drawn to these figures, it could mean you will also be drawn to work in a priestly or pastoral role.

Morganna le Fay

She is the legendary British Soul Midwife – half human and half fairy – who worked with the Grail energy, King Arthur and his lineage in the Isle of Avalon. She is still seen in her boat at the solstices, gathering the souls of the deceased. Her guidance is strong, pure and enchanting, and she has an affinity with mystical traditions, ritual and celebrancy.

The Northern Lights

The Labrador Inuit have an ancient myth that the northern lights are spirit torches lit at the end of each day to guide the dying home.

Modern Soul Midwives who feel drawn to work with the northern lights often have a gift for colour healing.

Peter Pan

Peter Pan is an iconic figure from children's fiction who represents an archetype working with the souls of children. The Lost Boys of this story bear witness to the work required to assist children, and those who are very young at heart, towards the light.

EXERCISE Learning from Sacred Traditions

You can develop your own insights into sacred traditions by studying the sacred texts, sacred music, prayers, customs and myths of other cultures as well as your own.

You could also:

- visit museums and study ancient sacred paintings

- explore other faiths to see how they support the dying

- talk to the elders in your community and ask them for their memories.

SUMMARY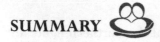

- Since the dawn of humanity, people have been caring for the dying and easing their transition.

- Only remnants of these ancient traditions have come down to us today, but we can benefit from their wisdom.

- Soul Midwifery is a modern, soul-based way of raising awareness of gentle dying methods and bringing compassionate loving care where it is needed.

- Soul Midwifery has now found its place: sitting side by side with modern medicine.

- People from all walks of life and of all ages are welcome to join the growing number of people practising Soul Midwifery (although if you wish to offer your services as a professional, fee-earning Soul Midwife, you will need to be properly trained, insured and mentored).

- An affinity with a certain tradition or archetype can be a clue to gifts, skills and potential ways of working.

- The love and care that we can give at the end of life are among the most precious gifts we can share with one another.

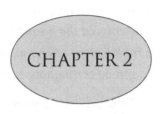

CHAPTER 2

SOUL MIDWIVES TODAY
AND WHAT THEY DO

'We're all here just turning into butterflies and flying each other home.'

SUCHI KUMAR

I am sitting with an elderly lady who is quietly passing away. She has been staring at the ceiling for many hours. Her tiny body, passive and fragile, is peaceful and very still. We sit together in companionable silence, listening to the dawn chorus outside.

I am intrigued by her intense concentration. What is she seeing? The face of her mother? A bright shining light? Or is she straining to hear ethereal sounds, perhaps? There are many stories about the visions that the dying experience when close to death. If the light in her eyes is anything to go by, she's enraptured and connected to something that is powerful and profound. There is no fear in her face; she is in no pain.

Her tiny hand feels quite cold and lifeless. But I can sense that a part of her is still fully functioning.

She has been like this for days, standing at some unknown threshold, looking as if she is tentatively exploring a new land. How long will she stay in this suspended state? No one knows. Everyone is surprised that she is still here.

Her name is Nora. She is 83, and a wife, mother, grandmother and great grandmother. She entered the hospice 10 days ago, on the very brink of death with a raging chest infection, the latest complication of the cancer that had spread throughout her body.

John, her husband of 61 years, hasn't been to see her. He can't. He just isn't ready. He stays on the farm and watches television all day, talking to no one.

Nora hasn't eaten or drunk anything for several days. But she is waiting – for as long as it takes. She won't go until John has been to say goodbye.

Two days later, Nora's daughter, Alice, arrives, bringing her reluctant father with her. He sits holding Nora's hand for several hours without removing his coat or woollen hat. I don't think he says a word, yet the room is filled with love. Eventually, after another hour or so, he goes off for a cup of tea and while he's away, Nora dies peacefully. She has chosen her time beautifully.

I open the window and feel her go.

As Soul Midwives we marvel at these mysteries of the dying hour and have deep insights into them. We know that as we watch, wait and listen, miracles happen. Many ancient societies regarded dying as the ultimate adventure in consciousness. Certainly there is something about the nature of death that sets the heart and imagination on fire. It touches the soul and sets the spirit free.

SERVICE

Sitting with someone who is close to the end is always a privilege, and the role of the Soul Midwife is one of service. We do not fix or rescue; we are there to support and to give tender loving care. Although many Soul Midwives do have a background in nursing, the majority are complementary therapists and counsellors, or just ordinary people who want to serve.

At the simplest level, Soul Midwives sit and keep someone company in the long dark hours which so often occur at the end of life. We will be there for as long as is needed, often standing in for friends or family to give them a rest, or becoming a special friend if there are no real ones. But at the other end of the scale, we are highly skilled energy medicine practitioners with a precise knowledge of the dying process. Many of us are also experienced holistic therapists, counsellors and celebrants. There are many different ways of practising the craft of Soul Midwifery, and we each bring to it our own talents and skills.

We support our dying friends from diagnosis to death and beyond. Death is usually a slow and gentle unravelling process akin to birth labour. It can be characterized by a series of important stages. Soul Midwives can offer support throughout the process:

- in the pre-active stage of death, when the friend is still fairly well and able to make decisions about death planning
- during the four elemental stages of dying
- in the active dying stage
- at the point of death and afterwards.

THE PRE-ACTIVE DYING STAGE

Preparation

Soul Midwives often work with people from the point of diagnosis, when they are still feeling quite well but know they have an illness that will shorten their life. If the Soul Midwife can work with the friend at this early stage, the therapeutic relationship can begin before the difficult times. Having plenty of time also enables the friend to plan for the type of death they want. This can be a very empowering process. Together, Soul Midwife and friend can make an end-of-life plan which can become a flexible map for the future.

However, before we can discuss the fact that someone is dying (even if it is very obvious, i.e. they have been admitted to a hospice), we have to be sure that they have accepted that they are dying and are comfortable talking about it. This doesn't always happen. Sometimes it only arises in the final few hours before death. Whatever the timing, the friend must always be able to control the content and pace of the discussion.

Once the discussion has begun, the Soul Midwife may be able to introduce a different perspective. For instance, if a friend has faced the shock of being told that there is no further medical treatment available, gentle questions may offer a new approach:

- 'Are there any memories that you would like people to have regarding the way you approached your illness and death?'

- 'How do you hope to be remembered in the future?'

- 'How do you hope your grandchildren will remember you?'

In addition, one of the skills a Soul Midwife should have is facilitating and sometimes initiating difficult conversations, such as what to expect during the dying process.

At this stage Soul Midwives will also help the friend to create memories for their families, such as recipe books, family albums, collections of favourite personal anecdotes, songs, poetry and family histories. And whenever necessary, they will offer comfort.

Comfort

A good Soul Midwife knows how to comfort and help the dying person by anticipating how they are feeling on all levels (physical, mental and spiritual), as well as supporting the family gently and acting as a wise and tranquil companion and caretaker.

Helping friends relinquish their fear of dying is important work, and sitting with them for as long as it takes, holding hands and reassuring them that all is well, will go a long way to dissolving the anguish.

Spiritual Companionship

As well as sitting with the dying and offering one-to-one care, companion-ship and support, Soul Midwives also offer spiritual companionship.

Our definition of the word 'spiritual' is both loose and wide: we are non-denominational, multi-faith and work alongside the beliefs of the person we are caring for. If they have no beliefs, that is fine too. Soul Midwives should, however, have an understanding of the main wisdom teachings and rituals of the major world religions, as they will be caring for friends of all religions.

Whatever their beliefs, many dying people want to talk about the meaning of their life and death. Soul Midwives can help to ease emotional concerns by listening and participating in these conversations. They can also offer:

- support for the beliefs of the person they are caring for

- simple celebrancy at the bedside, such as blessings, prayers and anointing

- heart-centred focus on understanding the friend's family and relationship dynamics

- help in healing soul wounds – the scars on our psyche inflicted by life, and in some cases past lives.

Soul Midwives can also enter into conversations about spiritual ideas and, if asked, introduce the idea of working with guides/ancestors/ spiritual figures to assist their friend's inner resources.

THE ACTIVE DYING PHASE

Therapeutic and Holistic Care

Eventually the friend will move into the active dying phase, usually in the last week or final few days of life. When this happens, the role of the Soul Midwife shifts from pastoral care to therapeutic and holistic care.

At this time a Soul Midwife uses a detailed model of the dying process which gives an idea of the feelings that the friend might be experiencing, psycho-spiritually, emotionally and physically. An experienced Soul Midwife should be able to conduct a simple examination of the friend to see how they are progressing, and how best to help them during the final days.

Soul Midwives are skilled holistic practitioners for the dying and will use touch, sound, breathing techniques, essential oils, simple handholding and stroking to alleviate fear and pain.

I expect many people reading this book will have had the experience of witnessing a loved one dying, and will remember how it is the simple things that seem to bring the most comfort at the end: the presence of family and pets, their own bed, clean sheets, a bedroom with fresh flowers and a window open.

What people don't want is to have their peace disturbed by clattering machines, unnecessary medical checks and a loud television in the background. Good pain relief and symptom control are vitally important, but the comfort of simple contact, soft lights, gentle music and a friendly presence are also of huge benefit in helping the dying to become less fearful and more accepting of the process. Creating a good environment is vital wherever the death is happening, whether it is in a hospital or in someone's home.

Our needs become simple as we die. If you were dying, what would comfort you?

- Someone to hold your hand?

- Peaceful and quiet surroundings?

- Fresh air?

- Time to just *be*...?

- Minimal intervention?

- Soft lights?

- Gentle music?

- Someone with whom you feel safe?

- Someone who has plenty of time and who understands how you are feeling?

Offering any of these small things is so simple, but for someone who is frightened and in pain, it can completely change the way they face death.

Vigiling

In the very final hours, we may be called (often by absent relatives) to offer a simple bedside vigil. This is simply watching over the friend and holding a sacred space for them. It is heartfelt companionship in the last hours of life.

This is how one Soul Midwife described helping her uncle, who was resident in a local care home:

> *We absolutely loved Uncle Fred. We formed a rota of nieces and nephews as well as his wife and four sisters to sit with him. We were all with him from after lunch on Monday until he passed away at 5 a.m. on Wednesday.*
>
> *We sat around his bed, talking and telling stories. We recounted all the family events that we could think of and laughed at some of the amusing memories. We weren't noisy, but we weren't quiet either.*
>
> *During the night, when I could see him struggling, I held his hand, along with Jane, his wife. We both talked him through a walk around his precious garden, smelling the flowers and feeling the breeze.*
>
> *Even though he was very much in and out of consciousness, we could feel him listening and we knew that he was very comforted by us being there, and he died with a lovely smile.*

We can help people make the transition, even when they aren't conscious. Gabriella Stevens is a Soul Midwife in her early thirties. She was called to an intensive-care unit to visit a man called Brian as he lay in a coma following a severe heart attack.

Brian had been there for five weeks. He had never regained consciousness. Eventually the family was given the tragic news that even if he woke up, his brain would be irreparably damaged. After agonizing discussions, the decision was made to switch off his life-support machine.

Gabriella was asked by Brian's wife, Claire, if she would anoint him and perform a small blessing ceremony releasing him and surrounding him with love as he died.

I used my singing bowl to create a sacred space, asking for the blessing of Brian's guides and angels to help us all. We played soothing music and dimmed the lights and his family sat around his bed.

With Claire's blessing, I ran my hands over his heart and chest and could feel the dense area which had been damaged by the heart attack. Already I could feel that life had truly left him. An aspect of him was somewhere else, although a tiny silver-like thread remained. He seemed suspended between two points.

I gently closed his chakras one by one, starting at the bottom and working my way up to the crown chakra. When I placed my hands above his head, I picked up his soul signal, which I felt like a pulsing throb pushing upwards.

As the machines were switched off, the silver thread connecting his spirit and soul thinned out and effortlessly pulled apart. It was a very sacred moment. We all felt him look down and hesitate for a split-second before expanding and bursting into a sphere of light.

Then there was a whoosh of energy. Everyone in the room felt it. There was no doubt at all that he had gone, and that the time was exactly and divinely right.

AFTER-DEATH CARE

In this hectic world, not many people have the time to devote themselves to caring for the recently dead, but it is a part of Soul Midwifery which is growing, as more of us begin to feel that there is a small interlude before a friend truly departs.

We always light a candle for our friends who have died, and often keep one burning for several days, sometimes weeks, until the need floats away.

The last three days after death are considered very sacred in many traditions, not least Christianity, in view of the story of Jesus' resurrection on Easter Sunday.

Even though many people die in busy places, such as hospital wards, where the body is removed quickly and dealt with, it still takes time for the subtle energetic aspects of transition to separate spirit and soul and loosen their connection to the physical world.

As well as looking after these energetic aspects after a friend has departed, Soul Midwives may be involved with practical tasks.

Preparing the Body

In the old days, the village wise woman would be called in to lay the body out in the front room of the home so that family, friends and neighbours could pay their last respects. Preparing the body for burial was the bread and butter of the Soul Midwife. This idea is currently seeing a revival.

If a patient dies in hospital, however, washing and preparing the body will be taken care of by the nursing staff. If a friend has died at home, the Soul Midwife will not usually be required to prepare the body before the undertaker arrives, but may be asked by the family to do so (*see pages 183–184*).

The Funeral

All religions have prayers and liturgy reserved for the dying, but ritual prayers and ceremony have also become the province of the Soul Midwife once again and we are often asked to create ceremonies and blessings. Some Soul Midwives are even taking on the role of the ancient priestesses and conducting funeral services as well. Some of the Soul

Midwives I have trained are funeral directors and celebrants offering a seamless service of care and companionship.

Gail Dyson, a Soul Midwife and funeral director in Manchester, is also a trained nurse and bereavement counsellor. She extends her work across the whole community.

Her unique funeral home is simply that: 'a home from home'. Instead of providing a sterile chapel of rest, she has created several individual 'bedrooms' where the deceased are tucked up in bed with pretty duvets and pillows. They are surrounded by candles and statues of the Buddha, which makes the atmosphere cosy and intimate.

There is no sense of the morbid here; Gail's office is a friendly place where people can walk in off the street and have a cup of tea and a proper conversation. She receives the deceased and their loved ones with as much tenderness and compassion as she would if they were special guests visiting.

When it comes to the funeral, the final celebration of the deceased person's life, she puts on a wonderful show – gleaming horses with plumes on their heads, brushed manes and a beautiful vintage hearse. She and her glamorous daughters dress in top hats and tails – every detail is taken care of and nothing is dull or routine.

Travelling with the Dead: Psychopomp Work

A psychopomp is a conductor of souls – a Soul Midwife or shaman who accompanies the dead on their last journey, at least part of the way.

Psychopomp work may involve being physically present when somebody dies and helping them to cross over there and then. Psychopomp shamans have the skill to accompany a dying person in their spirit body to show them the way into the beyond.

As Soul Midwives, we too may have to show lost or trapped spirits the way to the light. Even though their physical bodies have died, friends' energy bodies may still linger on the Earth plane and become 'earthbound'. There are various reasons for this, such as guilt, fear, religious conditioning, unfinished business or not enough spiritual energy to move to higher planes. The excessive grief of loved ones left behind, and their inability to let go, can also cause a spirit to become earthbound. And sometimes spirits don't even know they are dead.

When we work with earthbound spirits, we will spend time talking to them first. Some spirits need to be counselled to help them overcome a fear of annihilation, which is often the real reason for them not moving on. Soothing them and giving them confidence, as well as instilling trust in them and showing by example that there is nothing to fear, will in most cases be enough to convince them that it is safe to move forward. We offer all earthbound spirits love and compassion before asking that they be received by someone in spirit who loves them and will help them towards the light. We usually do this by sitting 'in circle' together or linking up at certain times when we can focus as a group and collectively hold the space.

Once the earthbound spirit is willing to move on, a portal to the beyond has to be opened for them to walk through. This may be done by the psychopomp through their own power or with the help of spirit guides.

The psychopomp may also be called on to help the spirits of those who are trapped in lower astral regions.

Helping trapped souls to move towards the light is an aspect of our work that is very sacred and should never be taken lightly.

MANY DIFFERENT ROLES

Soul Midwives are asked to help with many different aspects of dying, not just the obvious ones. The other day I worked with a woman in her forties who was dying from breast cancer. She was calm and accepted that she wasn't going to recover. She was a very organized person who had made a list of things to be completed before she went. This included writing letters to her children telling them about their childhood illnesses, and information such as when their first teeth had appeared, when they had first walked and what jabs they had had, as she knew her husband wouldn't remember. She then asked for help in framing some pictures that she had painted in her last months to give as goodbye presents to her godchildren. Finally, she directed me, from her bed, as I sorted out the linen cupboard. I filled several sacks with clothes for the charity shop while she sat up in bed giving me thumbs-up signs for 'Keep it' and thumbs down for 'Chuck it out.' We worked through everything on her list and when it was all done she went to sleep. She died a week or so later.

Another woman, very poorly, asked to be married at home in bed. I arranged this with the help of others, and she had a beautiful, simple wedding with wild flowers decorating her room. Her family and friends came and celebrated with her and her new husband. It was immeasurably moving, and bittersweet, as she died peacefully later that night, a bride for just six hours.

To sum up our many roles, these are the principles of Soul Midwifery:

THE 12 PRINCIPLES OF SOUL MIDWIFERY

1. To guide and support a dying person, and to help them achieve a loving, dignified and peaceful death.

2. To support and recognize the individual needs of the dying person, and ensure they feel loved and supported.

3. To create and hold a sacred and healing space for the dying person (whether in a hospital, a hospice or at home).

4. To respect and honour our friend's religious/spiritual/atheist/agnostic beliefs.

5. To work as non-denominational, multi-faith practitioners who do not impress their beliefs about life, death or the afterlife on their friends.

6. To listen, with empathy not sympathy.

7. To serve our friend, not aim to fix or rescue.

8. To be humble and work without ego.

9. To give healing, using sound, touch, colour or scented oils as required.

10. To keep a loving vigil.

11. To work with the spirit and soul of our friends at all levels and stages of transition.

12. To give loving care with a human touch.

We all have an ancestral memory of how to sit with the dying; it's in our bones. Whether we choose to become Soul Midwife or not in this life, it can be valuable to contact the 'inner Soul Midwife' and ask for any information that can help us now.

Access your inner Soul Midwife with the following exercise:

EXERCISE Contacting your Inner Soul Midwife

Concentrate on your breathing and relax. Fix your intention to connect with your inner Soul Midwife. Ask to be guided to discover knowledge that will help you now.

- What skills does your inner Soul Midwife teach?

- How do they work?

- Where do they work?

- What can they offer you in your work?

- What gift will they give you to take the work into your community?

SUMMARY

- Modern-day Soul Midwives are non-medical, multi-faith practitioners who support people facing the end of life.

- They offer holistic therapies such as massage, visualization, sound, essential oils, colour, Reiki and hands-on healing to create a calming, dignified atmosphere for the dying.

- They support the individual needs of the dying person and help them to fulfil their end-of-life wishes.

- They sit holding a vigil in the final hours of a friend's life and provide comfort and guardianship.

- After death they continue to offer their care and compassion in the form of prayer and connection for as long as is needed.

CHAPTER 3

THINKING OF BECOMING A SOUL MIDWIFE?

'If you help only one soul to find itself, if you comfort only one mourner, if you heal only one sick person, then the whole of your earthly life is justified. How privileged you are to be aware of the tremendous power that is around and about you, that enfolds you, guards you, directs you and ensures that you will continue to unfold your latent divinity and the gifts which are your cherished possession.'
SILVER BIRCH

My phone rang. It was a call from someone I'd never met; her name was Jan and she was so breathless she could hardly talk.

'I've been given your name. I have cancer and I am very angry, but I will fight it. I don't do pain,' she hissed in a frightened voice.

The language and tone of that brief conversation gave me some useful clues.

When I got there, Jan was sitting upright in bed. She looked like a colourful yet furious scarecrow: dyed purple-red hair, bright red leggings over tiny stick-thin legs and a purple T-shirt that hung off her skeletal frame.

'What are you staring at?' she growled. 'Am I so grotesque? Come here, sit on my bed! Everything's gone wrong. It's like this: I can't get up today. I can't manage this any longer.' And then she started to sob hysterically.

I perched hesitantly at the side of the bed, saying, 'I am so sorry to see you're in pain. How can I help you feel more comfortable?'

'Don't you dare be sorry for me!' she snarled. 'Just do something!'

She waved her hands in the air, raged on and howled.

I reached out and put my hand on her foot. It was absolutely frozen. 'Would you like me to warm your feet?' I offered.

She nodded and told me where she kept her ballet socks. Before I put them on for her, she let me take one foot at a time and warm it in my hands.

Then she shifted and began to tell me her life story. It was a tale of selfishness, anger, unresolved relationships, dramas, disasters and many regrets, and now it was all too late. She was very ill and it was obvious that there wouldn't be time to bring resolution to her problems.

All I could do was listen and hold her feet. Gradually she calmed down, the crying softened and she morphed into a very fragile, brittle, frightened woman who was finding it hard to let go and was desperately looking for forgiveness. She asked me for some healing and asked if I would come every day until the end.

When I called back the next day, her doctor was fixing up a syringe driver with morphine. I arranged to call back later, but she died that afternoon.

The practice of Soul Midwifery may be bittersweet at times, yet the path is a joyous one. It's also open to everyone. Is it for you?

KEY REQUIREMENTS

If you intend to charge for your services and help people other than your family or close friends, you will need to complete supervised Soul Midwifery training and be insured to practise. In the UK many Soul Midwives are also checked by the Disclosure and Barring Service.

Bear in mind that becoming a Soul Midwife requires dedication, study, practical experience and a programme of personal development and spiritual exploration. Certain skills may also be helpful.

USEFUL SKILLS AND PROFESSIONS

The following skills or professions are very useful if you are thinking of becoming a Soul Midwife:

Skills

- good listening
- massage
- creative visualization
- aromatherapy
- counselling
- dream work
- music therapy
- mindfulness
- meditation

Professions

- reflexologist
- psychotherapist
- priest
- nun, monk, celebrant
- funeral home assistant
- companion/carer
- doctor
- nurse

The key attributes to being a good Soul Midwife, however, are simply love, integrity, compassion and impeccability. And if you are hearing a call to become a Soul Midwife you will almost certainly have skills that you may not even realize are special and relevant.

Antonia Rolls is a Soul Midwife and also an artist who tours the UK with an astonishing exhibition called 'A Graceful Death', which arose from the death of her partner, Steve, from liver cancer. She explains:

We Soul Midwives are passionate about our work and are longing to work with those facing the end of life. We know we can do it; we all feel the need to change the perception of death by making it part of life (which it is), talking about it, acknowledging it and helping to prepare for it. We have found, though, that all of us work in different ways for the same end.

For a while I was confused, feeling that I couldn't possibly do the work that the other Soul Midwives did, and I felt that what I had to offer wasn't good enough. I didn't know enough, I wasn't trained enough, I hadn't enough experience...

[But] this is a time to stop faffing, and... do what needs to be done, listen to things that need to be listened to and at all times 'go with' whoever is dying, as far as they want you to go, in order that their death is the best it is possible for it to be. That is all you need to start.

And a Soul Midwife is not just someone who sits with another as they are dying; a Soul Midwife can help at any time, for a brief moment or for as long as it takes, along the journey from diagnosis to death. As long as we are there when called and we do what is necessary and what we can for that person who needs us, we are Soul Midwives.

There are Soul Midwives who are deeply experienced and are in the medical profession. There are Soul Midwives who run funeral businesses, who manage care homes, who offer complementary therapies for end-of-life conditions, who do more spiritual and alternative treatments like shamanism and Angel Reiki. There are Soul Midwives who are looking for a path to follow and haven't found it yet, but are drawn to the work. There are Soul Midwives who volunteer at hospices, at care homes; Soul Midwives who are looking after family members, friends, friends of friends as they die, and there are Soul Midwives who teach and help other people start their journey of helping the dying to die. There are Soul Midwives who comfort someone sitting next to them at a bus stop and move on because that encounter was all that was asked of them. I had a Soul Midwife encounter once with a man with months to live as we sat at the optician waiting to be called for eye tests. It was all that was required, and he moved on.

As a Soul Midwife... I do whatever I can that works. I do arty things, and fun things, and mostly I just watch and let the friend take the lead – but I have no training, no qualifications, no idea... I can't do alternative medicine, I can't chant and do singing bowls, and I don't know how to get someone off a bed and into a coffin... [But] it doesn't matter if I can't channel angels, or put in a drip successfully, or tuck someone neatly into a coffin so that they don't sit bolt upright after a quarter of an hour. It does matter that we do what we do well, and that we take inspiration from other Soul Midwives.

Sometimes when I look into the eyes of other Soul Midwives I see that they too [once] thought the whole area was full of things that they were not and we've all realized that we are absolutely fine.

We want to pool our resources and to support each other as we work, in our own way, to the same end: helping the dying to live well till they die, and to die as well as they can.

INITIAL CONSIDERATIONS

If Soul Midwifery is seriously calling you, there are several issues to consider, and working through the following exercise will help you to evaluate whether it is the right step to take.

EXERCISE **Is Soul Midwifery for Me?**

Think deeply about the following questions:

- Why are you drawn to this work?

- How do you respond to being with vulnerable people who may be in distress?

- How do you cope with being overwhelmed and exhausted – physically and mentally?

- How do you cope with witnessing difficult situations?

- Have you ever spent time with a dying person? If so, what did you learn from the experience?

- Have you lost anyone very close to you, and if so, how have you dealt with it?

- Have you developed a high level of personal integrity and impeccability in your daily life?

- Can you keep your mind and heart focused when you are tired, distracted and stressed?

- Are you squeamish?

- Have you (as far as you can assess) cultivated balance and awareness and an ability to step back and see the bigger picture?

- What are your beliefs about what happens after death?

- Could you become a spiritual companion to someone who is dying?

- Are you able to practise constant loving-kindness and compassion, with all that entails, even when you are confronted by people who challenge and hurt you?

- Can you work with the intense emotions of a frightened dying person at the same time as dealing with the emotions of other people (i.e. families)?

- Are you mentally and physically well?

- How strong is your own energy field?

Set aside a meditation/retreat day for yourself in order to reflect on the issues involved in becoming a Soul Midwife.

You will need to find or create a quiet space where you won't be disturbed. Create a sacred space (*see pages 86–95*), drink plenty of water, eat simple food such as soup, fruit and raw vegetables, and leave behind all distractions such as mobile phones.

Ask yourself:

- 'Why am I drawn to this work?'

- 'Whom will I serve?'

- 'How will I serve them?'

SKILLS REMEMBERED?

If you are drawn to this work, it may not be the first time. Many Soul Midwives have past-life memories of this work.

When one of my advanced groups worked with the ancient sacred oil spikenard we slipped into an intriguing group past-life experience. A dozen or so of us remembered in great detail our work within a monastic order at Abbotsbury in Dorset.

Abbotsbury is a beautiful village very close to the sea. It is famous for two things: a fourteenth-century chapel dedicated to St Catherine, which is perched high on a hill overlooking the village, and a famous swannery, which was established by Benedictine monks who built a monastery at Abbotsbury during the 1040s.

We could remember inhabiting a huge stone building which was our hermitage. Within the grounds was a lake fed by the still, fresh waters of the Fleet, a large, long freshwater lagoon which lies parallel to Chesil Beach. It seemed that we were Druid priestesses who had settled and worked there long before the Christian monks arrived and built their abbey. The area was hallowed and filled with healing energy. I have since learned that the Rose ley line, which runs from Rosslyn, south of Edinburgh, and carries the energy of the divine feminine, comes through Abbotsbury.

We had been part of a larger order of Celtic priestesses who were based at Glastonbury and had links with Joseph of Arimathea, Mary Magdalene and the Essenes. There were never more than 13 of us and we were easily recognized by our teal blue woollen dresses. Around our waist we carried tiny silver sickles hanging from a leather strap on our belts – an emblem of Soul Midwifery. The sickles were used to sever the spirit and soul from the physical body at death.

We could vividly recall receiving the dying in long, low flat-bottomed boats pushing their bows through the reeds of the lagoon. Once they had arrived, we took them into the sanctuary and prepared them for death. We used herbs (which were grown in the garden), music, song and sacred oils (including spikenard) to prepare the soul for its journey.

We were guardians of a small colony of swans which we regarded as living symbols of the soul. They served us in our releasing rituals and took the souls of the dead away across the water on their wide, feathered wings. They are still there, and are now a living colony of 600 wild birds.

Eventually we were ousted by angry monks, jealous of our skills. We were forced to scatter, taking our work to other places.

SOUL MIDWIFE PATHWAYS

Today there are three main pathways that weave together to form Soul Midwifery: healing work, the priest/priestess/celebrant path and that of the wise elders.

Healers

Soul Midwives with these qualities and skills perform holistic healing throughout the dying process. It may be offered as bedside work, distant healing, one-to-one, deep soul work and companionship to anyone facing the end of life.

This path attracts healers, Reiki practitioners, channellers, body workers, flower and gem remedy practitioners, energy practitioners, nurses, doctors, sensitives, empaths, Indigo and crystal archetypes, shamanic practitioners, homoeopaths, herbalists, clairvoyants, psychopomps, sound, colour and light therapists, aromatherapists, reflexologists, mindfulness practitioners, meditators and past-life therapists.

Priests/Priestesses/Celebrants

The priest/priestess/celebrant path relates to working as spiritual companions, thresholders (people who assist others in extreme states of mind, such as those who work on psychiatric wards), psychopomps and shamans. It involves soul work, journeying, working with soul wounds, grief and bereavement and deep inner work.

This path attracts celebrants, priests, nuns, shamanic practitioners, thresholders, lay chaplaincy, multi-faith ministers, ritualists, humanists, spiritual companions, past-life priests and nuns, mediators, counsellors, psychotherapists, clairvoyants, members of organized religions, and people with a strongly defined faith such as Quakers, Buddhists, Catholics and Anthroposophists.

Wise Elders

The wise elder Soul Midwives are earthy and practical. They are reliable, good at organizing, cooking meals, filling the kettle, tidying the sick room, walking the dogs, buying food, sitting and just being available. They are good listeners, a warm shoulder to cry on, a person to laugh with and share stories. They are usually good at creating memory work. These are salt-of-the-earth Soul Midwives with endless reserves of love and patience. They will sit for as long as it takes at the bedside of a dying person with a cup of tea and a warm heart.

This path appeals to sons and daughters, mothers and fathers, grandmothers and grandfathers, care workers, companions, death planners, educators, trainers, wise women and men, Soul Midwives already working within mainstream institutions such as palliative care, nurses and auxiliary carers, physiotherapists, occupational therapists, storytellers and teachers.

Psychopomps

Many Soul Midwives are also psychopomps, working with the souls of people after death for as long as is needed. This is a growing part of the work, and working with our friends after death, and continuing our love and care for them for a short time after death, has now become standard.

Psychopomp Soul Midwives may also work specifically with those who have died following large disasters such as tsunamis and earthquakes, people who have committed suicide and souls who are stuck in the astral realms.

GAINING EXPERIENCE

In practical terms, it may be difficult to gain experience of sitting with dying people unless they are close friends or relatives, or unless you are there in a professional role, as they are quite rightly protected from unnecessary intrusions. However, if you are taking your first steps along the Soul Midwife path, some Soul Midwives may let you shadow them during their visits.

To mentally explore what it would be like to be a Soul Midwife meeting a friend for the first time, why not try the following exercise?

EXERCISE **A Taster of Soul Midwifery**

Imagine that you have been called to sit with a neighbour who is dying.

- How would you mentally prepare yourself before walking into their room?

- How would you greet them?

- What sort of conversation might you have with them?

- What do you instinctively feel you could do to help them?

- Are you comfortable touching someone you don't know?

- How do you feel when you are with someone who is very ill?

- Are you easily embarrassed or made squeamish by bodily functions and outward sign of illness (such as catheters or unpleasant smells)?

- What skills do you have for comforting someone who is frightened or in pain?

FAQs

The following frequently asked questions should be of further assistance in helping you decide whether to become a Soul Midwife:

❧ *'Do I need to have medical qualifications to train as a Soul Midwife?'*

'No. Soul Midwives are non-medical helpers working alongside and in co-operation with the existing medical team. Soul Midwives come from all walks of life, including teachers, veterinary assistants, healers, undertakers, air hostesses and even rock stars! We are there to provide comfort, love and support – it's as beautifully simple as that.'

❧ *'I am a spiritual person but not religious. Does this matter?'*

'Not at all. We work with the beliefs of the people we are serving and help them in whatever way comforts and sustains them. Soul Midwives come from many faiths, including Anglican, Catholic, Buddhist, Quaker and Pagan. Many of our friends have no belief in anything at all. If this is the case, we simply offer companionship.'

❧ *'Do you have to be able to sense energy fields or can this awareness develop through training?'*

'This ability usually develops after training and practice. Even people who think they have no sensitivity in this way are very surprised by how quickly they are able to sense energy fields once they have been shown how.'

❧ *'I would like to be a spiritual companion Soul Midwife but am not drawn to doing hands-on bedside work. Is this possible?'*

'There are many ways to offer your services as a Soul Midwife and we each develop our own skills. If spiritual companionship and deep listening are your gifts, just specialize in those.'

❧ *'Can I charge for my work?'*

'Yes. Most Soul Midwives charge an hourly or block rate for their time, which is usually in line with local rates for services such as massage or counselling. Some workplaces, such as care homes, pay a retainer for Soul Midwives to come in as required.'

❧ *'I only want to volunteer my services. How would I go about doing this?'*

'Some Soul Midwives volunteer their services within small groups or organizations. These may include church groups, elder women's groups and rural community day centres.'

❧ *'My aunt and sister died last year and I was very involved with their passing. I still cry every day over how meaningful being with them was. I would like to be a Soul Midwife to help others.'*

'I would recommend leaving a gap and taking some time out for a while before considering this training. Your own grieving needs to be complete before you are able to help others.'

❧ *'How and where can I train?'*

'The Soul Midwives School runs practitioner training courses, advanced training and a variety of one-day courses for Soul Midwives. There is also a distance learning programme for those who are overseas and professional courses for those working in hospices, care homes and hospitals. (*For more details, see Resources, pages 250–258.*)

WHY DO WE NEED SOUL MIDWIVES?

Finally, we might want to consider the many different reasons why we need Soul Midwives:

- ✺ On a practical level Soul Midwives enable people to experience the deaths they would like to achieve.

- ✺ They are experienced guides, therapists and facilitators who understand the dying process and assist the dying on a deep and personal level.

- ✺ They are experienced in the spiritual, emotional and psycho-spiritual aspects of dying.

- ✺ They are also educators teaching people about death and dying.

- ✺ Soul Midwives are often the linchpins of local compassionate community initiatives.

- ✺ Soul Midwives can assist friends to shed their emotional baggage and soul wounds before they die so that they can cross the sacred threshold and move towards the light.

- ✺ On a spiritual and esoteric level, Soul Midwives prepare people for the great leap of consciousness that is transition.

- ✺ A Soul Midwife will literally midwife the soul, bringing it to birth on the next level.

AFFIRMATIONS

If you decide that you would like to explore Soul Midwifery on a deeper level, use this simple affirmation to acknowledge your readiness to begin the process:

'I open my being to the highest source and all aspects of the divine. I honour the journey that has led me to this point, enabling me to know who I am. I ask for love and compassion to assist me in helping others along their final journey.

Following in the footsteps of the wise elders who have practised this sacred art before me, I ask to be shown where my work may be done. I offer unconditional support, love, connection, depth and companionship to those who ask me to help them as they cross the sacred threshold.'

SUMMARY

- Soul Midwifery today is hands on and very practical, but also a demanding spiritual practice.

- Soul Midwives use many varied skills and talents in their work.

- Soul Midwifery is a craft, and each Soul Midwife brings to it their personal skills – no two Soul Midwives work in the same way.

- If you are drawn to Soul Midwifery, take the time to explore whether it is right for you.

❧ PART II ❧
CARING FOR
THE DYING

'The greatest privilege of a human life
is to become midwife to birth of soul.'

John O'Donohue

CHAPTER 4

HOW DOES IT FEEL TO DIE?

'Oh, wow! Oh, wow! Oh, wow!'

STEVE JOBS

Apple founder Steve Jobs' astonishment at facing death at the end of his journey with cancer in 2011 made headlines across the world and left millions of people wondering what he had experienced. What did he see? What did he realize? Were these the words of a rambling mind, muddled by drugs, or had he experienced a moment of enlightenment? We can only guess.

His sister, Mona, described more of Steve's final moments in the eulogy at his funeral:

...after a while, it was clear that he would no longer wake to us. His breathing changed. It became severe, deliberate, purposeful. I could feel him counting his steps again, pushing farther than before. His breath indicated an arduous journey, some steep path, altitude. He seemed to be climbing...

Then Steve uttered his last words and died in the presence of the people who were most important to him. His words are a wonderful affirmation of how curious and extraordinary the moment of death can be, and he planted in all of us the thought that death can be a peak experience, something unexpected – literally a 'wow' moment.

Despite modern medicine, death remains a mystery. How do we know what happens during the twilight before the last breath is taken? But if we are going to help people when they are dying, we need to understand what they are feeling.

This is how one of my friends, Carol, described her experience just hours before she died:

> I suppose this is dying. I'm feeling sick and exhausted; even my bed is uncomfortable now. I feel a detached numbness, as if my body doesn't really belong to me anymore.
>
> I could sleep for hours. If I go to sleep I don't think I will wake up now.
>
> I can't remember who I am. I am somehow watching myself go through this. But I am not frightened. I have done this before.

Dying is sometimes like this – we watch it happen as if we are actors in a play. But sometimes it comes as a complete surprise. As Eckhart Tolle describes it in *The Power of Now*:

> The tremendous shock of totally unexpected, imminent death can have the effect of forcing your consciousness completely out of identification with form. In the last few moments before physical death, and as you die, you then experience yourself as consciousness free of form. Suddenly there is no more fear, just peace and a knowing that 'all is well' and that death is only a form dissolving.

Death is indeed 'a form dissolving' – as the physical body dies, our lightbody shifts in vibration until the frequency is so high that we become pure energy once again. Soul Midwives are real midwives in the sense that they facilitate this birthing process.

HOW DOES IT FEEL EMOTIONALLY?

The moment of death may be liberating, but for many of us dying is a giant leap into the unknown. The process consists of three distinct psycho-spiritual phases:

- Chaos: When the discovery has been made that death is imminent, all safe boundaries are dissolved and there is often a feeling of emotional chaos.

- Surrender: After a period of fighting the illness, there comes a point of surrendering and going with the flow.

- Transcendence: A period – sometimes very brief, perhaps only during the last moments – of bliss and ecstasy as transition occurs.

Until that point, however, dying can be a time of fear. Many people say that given the choice, they would rather die suddenly and unexpectedly and thus avoid the fear and pain of knowing they are dying. Surviving family and friends may have many concerns, however. Did the person suffer? Did they have any last words? Could they have been spiritually prepared? When someone has died suddenly, family and loved ones often come to Soul Midwives with questions about those last minutes or hours.

What about an accidental death, such as being run over by a bus, or killed by a falling tree? Again, family and friends may be left wondering, but it may be comforting to know that on a soul level, the person leaves quickly in such cases. It's as if the soul steps aside before trauma strikes (avoiding soul fracturing).

If we have more time to contemplate our approaching death, however, this can be a time of bereavement – for ourselves and also for the life that we haven't lived. It is the end of our personal story. And, of course, it is a very painful time of having to say goodbye to everyone we are leaving behind. Not surprisingly, many of us feel angry, resentful, sorrowful and frightened as we die.

EXERCISE) **Leaving Life Behind**

Christine Longaker, spiritual care trainer and author, uses this exercise to show how it feels to leave life behind:

- First, I want you to think of the one person you rely on most heavily in the world, the person you love the most, the person you spend most of your time with. Now imagine that they have died.

- Next, I want you to think of another person in your life who is significant to you. Now imagine that they have also died.

- This may be harder, but now try to imagine that everyone you know and love and spend time with has died.

- Now that all your loved ones have died, imagine that your dreams have died too. Your plans for that holiday of a lifetime, the things you have always dreamed of doing, no matter what they are, imagine they are all now dead. Have you ever had to let go of a dream? If so, you know the grief I am talking about, though even then you usually had new dreams and plans to make up for the ones lost. Now you have none. No future to dream of or plan for.

If you can successfully imagine all of that, you are the closest you can get to understanding the grief of someone who is terminally ill.

Remember the grief you felt when a loved one died in real life, whether that was a spouse, a sibling, a best friend, a parent, a grandmother or a favourite pet. And imagine amplifying that loss to the loss of everything in your life.

The grief of the dying is great. It is more profound than any of us can imagine until we are wearing those shoes.

As already mentioned, when people learn they are dying, they very often like to look back over their life. Here's an exercise to give you an idea of the emotions that might come up as you do this...

EXERCISE Looking Back...

Imagine you have been told you will die in three months' time. Think about the following:

- What are the areas in your life where forgiveness is needed?

- What is the meaning of your life and your soul purpose?

- Who are the people you love, and how might you be able to help them as you die?

- What things do you need to let go of?

- Can you forgive yourself for things you now regret?

SHIFTS OF VIBRATION

Both the emotional and physical aspects of dying relate to shifts of vibration. These shifts take place as each of the four elements (Earth, Water, Fire and Air) of which we are composed withdraws from our body for the last time. These stages may take place gradually, over a period of weeks, or merge into each other seamlessly over days or hours or even minutes. As each element withdraws, our vibration is affected and we energetically 'lose our equilibrium'. Death occurs when all the elements have withdrawn and the body is reduced to an empty shell.

I first encountered the idea that we are all composed of four elements during my early quest to discover the mysteries of dying, when I spent over a year studying with a Buddhist nun who instructed me in the Tibetan tradition. Each element is a waveform and has its own energy signature. Together, the elements are the building blocks that connect the lightbody to the physical body and anchor spirit into matter.

When we are healthy, all four elements drift in and out of our body and spirit in a constant flow:

- Earth: While we are healthy, the Earth element represents our vitality, stamina, physical strength, zest for life, eagerness, curiosity, appetite, courage, forward thinking, anticipation and centredness.

- Water: The water element links to our emotions – pondering, pensive, anxious, mysterious, questing, melancholy, fearful, worrying, soul-searching, soulful, intuitive, full of trepidation, reflection and withdrawal.

- Fire: Gives us anger, transmutation, irritability, flashes of intuition, brilliance, determination and drive.

- Air: Associated with thinking, intellect, detachment, innovation, absent-mindedness and memory loss.

Every one of our thoughts, emotions and physical actions has an impact on how the elements run through our body. For instance, if we are sad, the Water element will be dominant. If we are angry over something, then the dominant element will be Fire, and so on.

As each of the elements leaves our body, it has a physical, emotional and spiritual effect on us. If we can be supported through these shifts, we move through them in a seamless flow. If the energy becomes blocked, it manifests as either physical or emotional pain, so the key is to keep it moving.

One of the most important aspects of Soul Midwifery is recognizing these stages and supporting people through them. (*See pages 99–105.*)

AT THE VERY END

It can also help us to serve the dying if we can understand what they might be feeling or experiencing at the very end. Fortunately, many people who have had near-death experiences have described what this feels like and this is backed up by descriptions in ancient texts.

Before we die, we experience:

- a chill spreading up through the chakras

- a tugging sensation as the subtle bodies detach

- a sensation of rocking backwards and forwards

- snapping and tearing sounds as physical and subtle bodies part

- disorientation (not being sure where sounds, etc., are coming from)

- an altered sense of time

- a diminishing of the senses, starting with touch and followed by taste and smell, then sight and hearing

- loud buzzing noises

- bright lights or a tunnel leading towards a very bright light.

As we move out of the body we are able to look down and see our empty shell. We then enter a tunnel of light where we are greeted by loved ones or spiritual beings and are enveloped in the purest energy of love.

THE SEPARATION OF SPIRIT AND SOUL

Soon after clinical death, when the heart has stopped beating and the last breath has been taken, the final stage, the separation of spirit and soul, will take place.

To many people, spirit and soul are one and the same thing. However, Soul Midwives tend to see a distinction between the two:

- *Spirit:* The transitory and ego-based aspect of our personality, relating to who we have been in this lifetime. It is fused to the ego and drives us on, throughout our lives, in an upwards, soaring, expansive and spiralling motion. It finally disperses and vanishes into the Air element, dissolving at the point of death or soon after.

- *Soul:* Our eternal template – a map of everything we are and have the potential to be – the soul spans all time and eternity. It is the great 'I AM presence' of the mystics, the primordial image of who we are. Its nature is deep, solemn and permanent. It is immortal. It evolves in a downward, labyrinthine and circular movement, and after death it completes its evolution back to the source of all being.

The separation of spirit and soul is an energetic event which can be intuited and sometimes seen as the separation of a thin silver cord which spins from a centre point in the body in two opposite directions.

The spinning motion thins the cord, which dissolves and separates the spirit and soul. Once this has happened, transition has fully taken place.

In ancient times, some Soul Midwives actually participated in this separation by cutting or blowing the cord. Small sickle-shaped implements, feathers or simply the breath were used. Today, Soul Midwives just sit and hold the sacred space while this event takes place, honouring the sacred moment.

SUMMARY

- Dying is a process, not just a moment when the heart stops beating and the breath ceases.
- As death draws closer, the elements withdraw, in sequence, for the last time.
- As the elements withdraw, our vibration shifts.
- Clinical death is followed by the separation of soul and spirit.

CHAPTER 5

PREPARATION

'In the end, just three things matter:
How well we have lived;
How well we have loved;
How well we have learned to let go.'

JACK KORNFIELD

I am waiting for a heart transplant. I have been warned that I could die before a donor is found. I live alone and this could easily happen when I am on my own, at night.

So I want to prepare in case that happens. I really want to die well, to recognize if it's happening and to consciously awake. I don't want to be taken by surprise, or miss it through not being prepared.

You could say that I have become slightly obsessed with the anticipation of my own death. This might sound macabre, but to me it's a way of living with the inevitable and it gives me an action plan. I am no longer scared but actually curious to know how it all works out. I picture my death being a bit like catching a huge wave and then surfing it. This is definitely a moment to practise for.

Surprise, surprise, since I've begun meditating on what will happen, I have connected with something huge – some sort of source energy. And I know it's Me. I will actually never die. I will step onto the wave and ride it without the encumbrance of my physical body. How cool is that?

For me, this is a form of enlightenment; I am now seeing the light. I know I will survive my death.

When it eventually happens, I plan to enter a deep space and breathe in, breathe out, with love. I will feel gratitude and peace and my passing will be soft and graceful.

GEORGINA

If we can begin working with a friend when they have been recently diagnosed, this gives us the chance to develop a deep bond of trust. They are still usually living a normal life: working, looking after family and home. With their diagnosis of terminal illness, they may go into a state of great shock and anxiety. This also links with the psycho-spiritual 'chaos' stage, where everything predictable and stable is in flux. There may be trauma, anxiety, anger and denial.

At this stage, we can come into a person's life and support them in practical and pastoral ways. As they adjust to their diagnosis, they may begin to form a plan of how they will navigate their illness. There will be treatments (or not) to be followed and choices to be made. This is a time when we will begin to work on end-of-life plans to facilitate the transition our friend desires.

LISTENING TO YOUR FRIEND

Companionship, good listening and quiet conversation are most important here. It is a good idea to talk to your friend privately as well as meet any caregivers to form a picture of how everyone is coping and how you can best support your friend.

When talking to friends and loved ones, it is a good idea to use 'open' questions (i.e. questions that cannot be answered with a simple 'yes' or 'no') to enable them to express themselves fully.

EXERCISE Learning to Use Open Questions

Here are some opening questions that you could use each time you greet your friend or carer/caregiver:

- 'How has your day been today?'

- 'How did you feel after our last session together?'

- 'How can I serve you today?'

- 'Is there anything causing you pain or anxiety?'

Remember to always greet your friend with a smile and a cheerful countenance. When someone is dying, their loved ones may find it difficult to be happy around them, and it makes your smiles all the more important. Loved ones may also feel uncomfortable when the friend wants to discuss death or the dying process, so it is especially important that a Soul Midwife allows the friend to voice their concerns and to be heard.

Always follow the friend's lead. If they talk about their impending death, either directly or indirectly through metaphor, go along with it. If they ask you if they are dying, be honest, but avoid a blunt 'yes' answer. You could reflect the question back and say: 'I don't know. What do you think/feel?'

A good Soul Midwife will listen not only to what is being said, but also to what is not being said. Encourage your friend to tell you their journey so far, particularly the moments that have been significant for them.

HOW TO BECOME A GOOD LISTENER

There are a number of points to remember when listening to your friend:

- Take the time to meet and greet your friend properly.

- Give your friend your complete undivided attention.

- Don't interrupt them or talk over them.

- Hold their hand (if possible) and maintain soft eye contact.

- Use 'open' body language, i.e. don't sit with your arms crossed.

- Lean slightly forward to show you are engaged and interested.

- Use gestures to show you are listening, and don't allow yourself to be distracted.

- Empathize, don't sympathize.

- Be patient and give them time to say what needs to be said. They may find it difficult to talk about certain issues or physically draining to talk at all.

- Listen with your *eyes*: non-verbal clues may affect the meaning of what your friend is saying, i.e. if they are clasping their hands this may indicate that what they are telling you is very emotional or painful for them.

- If you are unsure of what your friend is trying to communicate, try to clarify matters when they have finished speaking.

- Take a conversation slowly – not rushing to respond to what a friend is saying may give them the space to say more.

- Show acceptance.

ADDRESSING FEARS

Shallow reassurances and avoidance of difficult issues have no place in Soul Midwifery. If your friend has fears, encourage them to share them. If the fears can't be resolved, they can at least be heard – witnessed, in a sense – and perhaps in that way laid to rest.

Sometimes fears can be resolved: if there is fear of not being able to heal a family rift, for example, there may be the opportunity to do something about it. Even if not, it can be tremendously important for the friend just to tell their story.

The friend may express anxiety about finishing certain tasks. Ask them to tell you more. You may be able to help.

If someone is having real difficulties in letting go, help them to reflect on the innumerable deaths that we all encounter as we move through life – leaving behind our babyhood, our childhood, our teenage years and so on.

One of the commonest fears that dying people express is that they don't know where they're going. Many people fear that dying is like falling off a cliff into darkness. To counter this, one of the most valuable things we can do is to help our friends create a peaceful journey to a happy place where they can rest after death.

EXERCISE Going on a Journey

This is a simple but very important visualization that your friend can use in their final hours. This technique is very powerful, and really does help people who may have fears about letting go and surrendering to death.

You can guide your friend through the visualization to begin with, and later they can take themselves through it on their own. It can be a useful resource to draw on when faced with moments of pain or fear.

Imagine you are walking through a garden gate into a beautiful garden which has a winding cobbled path that leads to a gap in a wall.

Through the wall is a building made of glass and light. It is filled with roses of every colour imaginable: pink, red, dusky apricot, white...

You smell them one by one...

Or:

Imagine opening a small gate from a garden into a flower-filled meadow where butterflies are flying from flower to flower.

A grassy path winds towards a flowing green river.

You take off your shoes and feel the soft grass under your feet and hear the birds singing in the trees.

Many people also like to imagine a safe place or room where they will rest after transition. This imagined room can be very helpful for people who are frightened of being abandoned in the black unknown hole of death. Sometimes it is seen as a room filled with healing colours, light and music. It may have a wonderful view across an endless ocean or have a doorway into Paradise. Sometimes loved ones or pets are waiting there to escort the person to heaven.

One friend I worked with was a passionate dog-lover. She created a story where all the dogs she had ever loved would be waiting for her in a little house in the middle of some woods. As she got closer to death, she knew that each of her beloved pets would be waiting on the other side of the threshold. As she was dying, she murmured that her favourite 'soul' dog, Carl, a scruffy rescue collie, had come to take her home.

Creating a narrative like this can be one of the most important aspects of the pre-active phase and is very deep and profound work in itself. You can really see the benefits of it when you are sitting with someone who is in their final hours, not able to speak but still able to hear. You can see them following their imagination and letting go of their fear.

ACCEPTANCE OF MORTALITY

These conversations and visualizations can only happen if the friend has accepted that they are dying and is comfortable in talking about it. This doesn't always happen, and then maybe only just before death.

Remember to always let the *friend* direct the content and pace of the discussions. You can, however, gently guide friends to think about their mortality. This can be done in many different ways. I was sent this series of prompts by a colleague many years ago. I don't know who originally created it, and it has been adapted over time, but I find it very useful as a tool for beginning potentially difficult conversations:

- What keeps you from standing in your power and manifesting who you are?

- Who are you truly?

- Who are your allies?

- What gives you strength when you are in the deepest, darkest despair?

- How do you call on this strength?

- What do you wish to call into your life? What do you wish to integrate and accept?

- What parts of your life are you ready to release or bury?

- What are the obstacles, inner or outer, which keep you from letting go?

- What are the attachments in your life, and how do they control you?

- What attitudes, belief systems or habits no longer serve you? What are the shadow aspects in your life?

- What do you really fear and resist?

- Do you hear a calling for a new and different life?

- How will you answer that call?

PREPARING TO DIE

Once a friend has accepted that they are going to die, you can work together on end-of-life planning. This may evolve over many weeks. Many people find it an inspiring and empowering process. It brings a sense of creating something very important and meaningful. It's a time of 'putting their house in order' in both practical and personal terms.

As Dee Dade, a Soul Midwife and bereavement counsellor based in Dorset, says:

> People still imagine that they are going to die naturally, probably in their sleep. It simply doesn't occur to them that it just doesn't happen like that to most people these days.
>
> A hospital or hospice is a completely alien environment and beginning treatment and starting new drugs can be very disorientating right at the end of life. Most people aren't able to say, 'No, I've had enough', partly because of the drugs and partly because they are frightened and overwhelmed.
>
> If ideas and preferences have been written in advance, then the Soul Midwife can be a very helpful advocate at the end of life.

To get an idea of what to consider in end-of-life planning, try the following exercise.

EXERCISE How Would You Like to Die?

Think about the following:

- What kind of music, or what songs, would you want to hear?

- Would you prefer silence?

- Who would you like to be with you?

- Would you like any healing, stroking or talking?

- What spiritual figure or guide may be there for you?

- Which of your loved ones might be waiting?

- Have you imagined a place where you can rest and heal after you have died?

- What does it look like?

Putting the House in Order

There may be many practical issues to consider. These include:

- financial considerations, such as making a will

- advance care directives such as a Living Will

- arrangements for the care of pets if the friend is hospitalized, or when death occurs

- identifying a network of friends and helpers to help with practical issues such as transport to hospital appointments

- helping to contact people with whom your friend may have lost touch.

EXERCISE Creating an End-of-Life Plan

It is useful to work together to formulate a specific end-of-life plan. The following questions can help with this. They are always for the friend to answer, based on their own set of values and beliefs.

- Where would you like to die? At home, in hospital or in a hospice?

- How involved in your care and medical decisions do you hope to be?

- Do you want to remain lucid at all times and be able to make decisions?

- Would you prefer medical information to be given to a partner or a relative? (Some people may not wish to find out that they are dying from a member of the medical staff but from someone closer to them. They may also wish to discuss it on a spiritual level with someone else.)

- Would you like any religious ceremonies or rituals prior to death?

- Would you like singing, chanting or poems/prayers spoken out loud?

- Would you like to be anointed, or to receive healing or any other therapies close to death?

- Who would you like to have with you – or not have with you?

- Are there any outstanding issues, emotional or financial, to be resolved?

- How long would you like to be left after you have died and before you are removed and prepared for burial or cremation?

- What sort of funeral would you like?

~~~~~~

There is an example of a simple end-of-life plan in Appendix I.

SPIRITUAL COMPANIONSHIP

The end of life often opens up questions about the greater meaning of life and our part within it. Soul Midwives are non-denominational, but spiritual companions in the very widest sense, embracing every belief or no beliefs at all. Many of the friends we help have no spiritual interests. A starting point with someone who requests spiritual companionship can be as simple as helping them make a connection with their inner divine self and remembering their connection with something greater than themselves.

Dream Diaries

Dreams recorded as text, drawings, paintings, etc., or via an audio recording device, can be very helpful pre-active work. Many people find that working with their dreams is a gateway to exploring inner issues.

Memory Work

At this time our friends often want to reflect on the story of their life and how they lived it, and to leave something behind for their loved ones. Memory projects may include:

- memory boxes

- recipe books

- CDs, such as reading nursery rhymes for grandchildren

- video clips

- songs

- poems

- painting

- pottery

- plaster casts of hands.

Here again, people enjoy the process.

THERAPEUTIC WORK

As we work with friends, we can see them beginning to pull away from life, even though death may still be some way off. Sometimes we notice a change when we haven't seen an old friend or relative for some time. Somehow, without being able to put a finger on it, we can see that they are somehow different – a little older, perhaps frailer. Here are some suggestions for 'tuning in' to understand what may be happening for them:

- Concentrate on really listening to what they are saying – there may be hidden clues as to how they are feeling deep inside.

- Give some very simple healing. It can be as easy as stroking an arm or hugging.

- Follow your intuition and be guided as to how you might be able to help them.

- Don't feel you have to fix or change anything – just be yourself and allow the space to open up.

During this stage we also introduce our friends to therapies such as massage, gentle touch, Reiki, meditation and working with sound. (*For more on these, see pages 124–125.*)

Soothing Soul Wounds

Soul wounds are the scars left by this life, and in some cases past lives. Soul wounds don't respond to morphine. They probably can't be healed completely in the short time that we spend with someone who is dying, but they can be soothed by love and brought into the light and honoured.

Soul wounds can hamper the seamless flow through the transitional phases of dying, and one of our roles as Soul Midwife is to work with them in whatever way we can.

They may manifest in the following behaviour:

- frequent and excessive anger

- excessive and irrational fears

- self-medication with the abuse of prescription drugs, street drugs, alcohol and pornography

- sexual addiction, food addiction, shopping addiction

- compulsive dishonesty; constantly telling half-truths or untruths about one's life and circumstances

- the need to control

- excessive anxiety

- feelings of suspicion and distrust

- strong feelings of being unloved or unworthy

- an inability to love and enter into deep relationships.

The important things that we need to remember about soul wounds are that:

- They are real.

- They may be extremely painful.

- They are often emotionally and spiritually crippling.

- They frequently distort friends' view of reality.

- They create painful and fractured relationships which will often affect the whole family.

Sometimes a soul wound is very obvious, but sometimes there is a complicated overlap of many different wounds.

Your friend's soul wounds may also trigger a response in you, forcing your own wounds up to the surface. The key is to know yourself and know your own wounds. How can you recognize them? Think for a moment. What bothers you when you are tired? Or depressed, or feeling anxious? This probably points to your own soul wounds.

One of the best ways of dealing with soul wounds is to recognize them, acknowledge them and then love them and let them go.

Here is an affirmation for acknowledging your own soul wounds:

'Even though I feel abandoned and unsupported at times, I recognize that this is just a part of who I am. I recognize the fact that these feelings can be challenging, but they don't undermine my core wellbeing or my ability to help others.'

RECORD KEEPING

It is very important to keep a written record of the time spent with your friend. Not only does this give you documentation to refer back to, it can also be a record of safe practice.

You may wish to record the following:

- up-to-date contact details of your friend and their family

- the dates and duration of your meetings

- your friend's expectations (this will help you to assess whether you are meeting those expectations)

- any home-care advice you give (i.e. diet and relaxation exercises) and whether it has been followed

- how the friend is feeling

- the effects of any treatments – both positive and negative

- whether (and how much) the friend has paid you for your time.

Adding brief notes at each session will ensure that you continue to work with your friend and meet their expectations.

SUMMARY

- While not always possible, it is ideal if you can create a bond of trust and friendship with your friend in the pre-active stage.

- Deep listening skills will enable the relationship to develop.

- Addressing fears and anxieties will speed acceptance.

- It is helpful to create a personal guided visualization to ease your friend through pain, or the final stages.

- End-of-life plans can provide a valuable guide to friends' wishes.

- Memory work and projects can be prepared now – recipe books, photo albums, poems, sound and video recordings...

- Keep accurate records of your friend's progress.

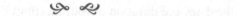

CHAPTER 6

LISTENING WITH THE HEART, SEEING WITH THE HANDS

'And now here is my secret, a very simple secret: it is only with the heart that one can see rightly; what is essential is invisible to the eye.'

THE LITTLE PRINCE

When I was a child, meeting new people and going to new places was torture. Even normal activities, such as school and ballet lessons, and childhood treats like birthday parties and family outings were events I dreaded.

It wasn't that I was shy – far from it. The problem was that I was super-sensitive. On every level I could see and hear and sense so much information that I was always overwhelmed by everything around me. Not only could I sense things and experience premonitions, but if someone held my hand or sat me on their knee, I could sense their energy and read their thoughts. And these weren't always pleasant.

I began to be very wary of adults, especially those who said one thing but meant something entirely different. There weren't many people I could trust completely or feel safe with.

Besides reading people and knowing whether they were telling the truth, I could also smell if they were ill, even if the illness hadn't manifested yet. This was very upsetting, as I didn't have a way of dealing with the situations I could see happening to them in the future. I remember hearing an aunt talking about the cruise of a lifetime she was going on in a few months' time and knowing that she'd have a heart attack. She died on the ship at Southampton half an hour after boarding.

Houses, places, even cars made me fearful. Staying with school friends was impossible. While everyone in the house slept, I'd see things hovering in the shadows and have innocent conversations with the family's 'dead' relatives (I didn't realize that they were dead). After a while, not surprisingly, parents began to discourage their children from asking me back for tea. I was always very relieved. Home was best.

Gradually I learned to disguise my peculiarities. I was bright and outgoing and became a very skilled chameleon. I also learned to keep quiet and not to speak my truth.

Like many sensitive children, I was often ill. I suffered sudden soaring temperatures, vomiting, body rashes, strange infections, raw patches of weeping eczema and severe allergies, especially to medicines and certain foods.

In my teens, I slowly learned to cure myself of many of these problems by adjusting the amount of energy I created in my body. After a time, I realized that I could do this for others.

I come from a family of sensitives and healers, although none of them are comfortable sharing or using their gifts.

In my mid-forties, I experienced a huge power surge in my abilities. With no warning, I woke up one morning after a normal night's sleep and felt as if I had been completely rewired – or, to look at it differently, wired up properly for the first time in my life! It was as if the volume dials on all my senses had been turned to full. Everything danced and pulsed with light. New colours leapt in vivid arcs before my eyes, and I seemed to have developed some form of X-ray vision. With my inner vision, I could clearly see through cross-sections of solid matter, as well as see multi-dimensional layers around people. I could see the weaving energy currents of crystalline light that sit layer upon layer on top of the physical body. For the first time, I was seeing the human energy field – the lightbody.

In the background, I could hear a constant chat – the chat-chattering of hundreds of voices muttering across telephone wires. My fingers tingled and vibrated, and I could move energy around me with my hands.

I felt as if I had burst out of my body, shed several skins, flown backwards and forwards through a few time zones and then been slammed back in again.

Thankfully, I knew a little about what could happen during shamanic initiations and also about Kundalini awakenings, which can occur without warning, so I knew that I probably hadn't gone completely 'mad'! Also, I was sure, without any doubt at all, that I was remembering something that I had once known. It was as if a missing part of me had returned.

As luck would have it, several extraordinary teachers synchro-nistically showed up in my life and I was guided through this peculiar, and at times harrowing, initiation. Then, at last, my real work began.

SEEING THE LIGHTBODY

Many years after this strange initiation, when I had grounded my experience and was beginning to develop my work with the dying, I came across the work of two very different artists, both visionaries, with a form of X-ray vision.

The first one, Alex Grey, is an American who leads a sophisticated New York City life, and the other, Joska Soos, was a humble peasant shaman from a village in Hungary, yet both have been able to enter altered states and see and paint the lightbody.

Alex Grey is revered for his powerful work, which began after he took LSD. The drug expanded his clairvoyant sight and prompted a deep understanding of energetic anatomy. He spent five years working in the Anatomy Department at Harvard Medical School, studying the body and preparing corpses for dissection. As a result of his extraordinary abilities, he was then invited to work at Harvard's Department of Mind/ Body Medicine, where the human energy matrix and its various subtle healing energies have been tested in a series of scientific experiments.

Healers the world over have praised Grey for the way he exactly captures complex etheric anatomy. His famous picture of a dying man with a plume of energy leaving the crown chakra, moving upwards towards a source of light, is exactly what I have seen when supporting friends at the Fire stage of transition (*see pages 103–104*).

Joska Soos was an artist of a very different type. He was a very powerful shaman born into the de Basca shamanic clan who developed the gift of seeing human energy after communing with what he described as trans-dimensional 'light-sound' beings.

He developed his super-sight while working as a miner. The total darkness and silence he experienced deep underground enabled him to sense certain high vibrations and expand his consciousness. When a mining shift ended, he would stay underground for an hour or so, completely alone in the darkness, in order to commune with the frequencies.

Soos said that after his initial encounters down the mine, the light-sound beings he met there began to appear when he shamanized for people. They taught him how to work with their high vibrations and expand his consciousness. They always gave him knowledge and energy, but their frequency was so high that he was prevented from getting too close to them by an invisible field. When he accidentally broke through the field once, he was struck down as if by a bolt of electricity, which put him into a deep coma for six hours.

Soos saw the lightbody as a primal yet complex pattern of muted geometric forms very similar to crop circles. His paintings – and there are hundreds of them – capture the individual 'soul essence' of people. Their sacred simplicity reduces many people to tears and brings a sense of recognition.

Soos also worked with singing bowls. These can increase our sensitivity by helping us resonate with wavelengths that are connected to different levels of consciousness. We know that in the normal waking state the brain produces beta waves, but it has been discovered that when we meditate or listen to specific singing bowls, it switches to the alpha frequency. This makes us feel calm and mindful, and makes singing bowls potentially powerful tools of consciousness.

Dr Mitchell Gaynor, Director of Medical Oncology and Integrative Medicine at the Cornell Cancer Prevention Center in New York, has researched the healing effects of singing bowls. In a blind study, he noted a 50 per cent decrease in recovery time for cancer patients receiving chemotherapy when they experienced singing bowls regularly. He also found that introduction to singing bowls early after diagnosis greatly reduced anxiety and stress levels in his patients.

As well as using tools such as singing bowls, we all have a latent radar system for picking up other people's emotions, and we can also develop our sensitivity in order to sense physical and spiritual pain. This is what gives us all the capacity to become Soul Midwives.

In fact, developing sensitivity to energy is something that grows with the work we do. It also seems that one of the gifts of 2012 was that many people experienced upgrades in their capacity to see and feel on a higher level. We can use this in our energy work with the dying.

ENERGY HEALING

In the active stage of the dying process, Soul Midwives become companions, sitting at the bedside as the labouring begins and the four elements withdraw. Soul Midwifery at the bedside incorporates a variety of practices, and in many of them Soul Midwives are energy technicians, using their inner vision to read energy fields and perform energy healing.

Energy healing is a type of bodywork that uses hands-on techniques to restore balance to the electromagnetic field that surrounds a person internally and externally. Energy flows from the healer's hands to the individual, whose body receives it as needed. As healthy energy is restored, stagnant energy is released. Energy healing stimulates the body to reach its optimal level of balance in order to heal itself.

When performing energy healing on the dying, it is important to work at the level of the energy field, as it is deeper than the level of the physical disease that the person is dying from.

Touch itself heals through a direct link from the heart and the hands – it's a natural form of communication without words. Soul Midwives understand not to be anxious or hesitant about touching someone; we know our heart will guide our hands.

Simply sitting with someone and holding their hand creates a deep link and sends a message that we are treating them with tenderness and dignity. Quite often, dying and seriously ill people are only touched as part of a medical examination or for cleanliness purposes. People whose illness makes them look or smell unpleasant may become virtually untouchable for any other reason and can quickly feel very isolated and alone. Consequently, sitting with them and holding their hand, or gently rubbing their feet, can make a huge difference to their wellbeing.

If a friend has developed an unpleasant body odour, put tiger balm under your nose to help mask the smell. You could also try breathing through your mouth or sucking menthol sweets.

It is not appropriate to use conventional massage on people when they are dying – it is too strong and invasive. However, soothing touch (also known at Therapeutic Touch, Jam Che or Gentle Touch), Reiki or other forms of energy healing can provide healing with the comfort of touch. A simple and very gentle hand or foot massage with scented oils and creams can be very soothing. Washing or warming someone's feet with your hands is also a very nurturing and humbling act.

Occasionally, of course, people aren't comfortable with being touched in any way. Be very sensitive to this, as the friend may be past speaking and only able to convey their discomfort by tensing up or looking distressed. If someone doesn't look as though they are comfortable with what you are doing, *always stop*. Remember, you are not there to *help* but to *serve*.

Overall, energy work with the dying requires:

- setting a field and then working within it

- using the frequency of love as the 'intention' for the work

- tuning in to the lightbody

- using sound and light to clear energy blockages.

We do this by listening with our heart, seeing with our hands and understanding that the heart is the portal or gateway for the soul.

Very experienced Soul Midwives may even work in the dream state. This is the place we inhabit when we leave our body at night and expand into the astral realms. When we are dying, we spend more and more time there, especially when we are experimenting with how it feels to be out of our body. Working in the dream state is a very specialized form of healing that requires years of practice, and mentoring by someone already very experienced in the field.

Any form of energy healing with the dying takes dedication and patience – there are no short cuts. Developing the inner vision necessary usually requires having your own frequency expanded and attuned (similar to a Reiki attunement). If you haven't studied energy work, you will need some preliminary training in basic anatomy and physiology and healing skills before attempting any energy healing techniques.

There are several ways of doing this, including:

- studying spiritual healing

- studying Reiki

- taking a basic anatomy and physiology course.

(*For more details, see the Resources section.*)

If this feels a lot to take on initially, you can always investigate this aspect of Soul Midwifery when you feel it is right for you. In the meantime, you can always use soothing touch (*see page 84*) and colour therapy (*pages 122–123*), as these require no experience in energy work and can still provide great relief to your friends.

Once your friend has reached the active dying stage, however, first of all it is essential to create a respectful, soothing atmosphere, a sacred space or field that will help the dying person and honour the sacred act between you when you are performing healing or rituals.

CREATING A SACRED SPACE

As we die, the bonds that weave our body and soul together begin to loosen and detach. Very subtle changes in the senses occur to help us face these final changes. Part of the reason why dying people are so delicate and fragile is because their senses are unusually heightened. This means they are vulnerable to extremes such as bright lights, loud noises and uncomfortable surroundings.

Sacred space helps to detach the dying person from the outside world and all its noisy interruptions and distractions. It creates the ambience to allow the inner unfolding that takes place as the physical body diminishes and the soul strengthens.

What constitutes as 'sacred' will vary from person to person. In some parts of the world, the entire community focuses on creating a sacred space for a person who is dying. For example, Varanasi, the sacred Indian city situated on the banks of Ganges, is the most auspicious place for Hindus to die. By dying here, it is said, one has a good chance of breaking the cycle of life and death. So the whole city has been turned into a sacred space. Everyone who lives there respects and honours the dying in their midst. There are even special dying houses where people can take their loved ones and sit in vigil over them.

Size is irrelevant, though, and you can easily turn any small corner of a room or a curtained-off area in a hospital or hospice into a sacred sanctuary.

1. Preparing Yourself

Before opening a sacred space, you should:

- Clean yourself – either symbolically by meditating or by taking a bath and changing into fresh clothes. This helps you to become a clear channel for the energies.

- Drink lots of fresh water and refrain from alcohol for 24 hours either side of this work.

- Set your intention by emptying your mind and focusing on what you are about to do.

2. Preparing the Space

Space clearing is a simple ceremony to revitalize the energies that have become imprinted over time in the walls, furniture and other objects of a room. Energetically, everything that ever happens in an area becomes imprinted on that space, and this is especially true when dealing with the energies of illness and death. The residue of these energies ripples around the edges of a room and builds up, particularly in corners. This is why a room where illness has lingered can feel heavy and sticky. In hospices and hospitals, where many people have died, you can often sense a heavy blanket in the atmosphere which dulls the space. This can be cleared in several ways:

- Begin with a thorough cleansing. Apart from soap and water, sunlight and fresh air will help to remove any stagnant energy in the room. Fling open the windows and doors to get the breeze flowing through. Dust and wipe the furniture and sweep the floor. Make sure everything is neat and tidy. Negative energy loves the chaos of clutter.

- If cleaning isn't possible (perhaps the friend is using the room), try sprinkling salt into all four corners (salt is a natural cleanser, attracting and absorbing negative energy) and use sound (tingshas or singing bowls) in the corners to break up, disperse and move any stagnant energy lingering there.

- Then announce your intention. I like the boldness of something like,

    'I ask for the lightest and brightest aspect of divine love to fill this space in honour of my friend's passing.'

    or

'I call on my spiritual helpers and those of my friend to help me clear and purify this space.'

- You may, if you wish, call in the four directions (North, East, South and West) at this point and invoke the four elements (Earth, Air, Fire and Water) before you begin:

South, West, North and East,
Please hold this space in peace.
Earth below and sky above,
Please hold this space in Love.
CHARLOTTE GUSH

3. Purifying the Space

Using Aromas

Scent is evocative. Just smelling a beautiful flower, freshly baked bread or the first drops of rain after a hot summer's day can shift our mood dramatically. Different perfumes can make us happy and uplifted or reflective and tranquil. Indeed, smell is the only sense directly linked to the brain's limbic system, which controls memory and emotion.

Around 75 per cent of our emotions are thought to be generated by what we smell, so using scent can be a highly effective way of inducing states of tranquillity and peace. And certain aromas can enhance not just emotional wellbeing but physical healing too.

A study at the Christie NHS Foundation Hospital in Manchester in 2011 looked at the benefits of using aromasticks in people with cancer. Aromasticks are similar in design to vapour inhalers for cold relief. They contain essential oils and aim to help patients manage anxiety, nausea and sleep disturbance. In the study, 160 people used the aromasticks and 77 per cent reported at least one benefit from them.

Of the anxious patients, 65 per cent reported feeling more relaxed, and 51 per cent felt less stress. Of the nauseous patients, 47 per cent said that the aromastick had settled their stomach, while 55 per cent of the people who had sleep disturbances felt that the aromastick had helped them to sleep.

The fragrances of burning sage, incense, scented candles and fresh flowers all have a calming effect. Scenting a room will help carers and visitors too!

You might like to spritz the air with essential oils (*see pages 117–121*).

Depending on your tradition, you may also smudge the air with white sage bundles. These are available in many holistic shops and are very helpful for clearing the space – as well as creating a pleasant clean, woody smell.

When people are dying, their sensitivity to odours can be acute, however, so if the friend has a negative reaction, remove the fragrance immediately.

Using Sound

Using sound to cleanse a room can be very effective and uplifting. Tingshas, the ancient cymbals which are widely used in Tibetan temple ceremonies, are used for clearing and cleansing environments so that the area is once more 'open' and harmonious. Based on the principles of *feng shui*, tingshas and singing bowls can be used to restore vitality and harmony in energetically discordant areas.

Simply striking a bowl on its side with a soft mallet, and allowing the tones to circulate throughout the room, or ringing tingshas in each of the corners of the room, will be enough to remove stuck energy. Walk around the room, ringing the tones high up towards the ceiling and down close to the floor, paying special attention again to the corners and behind the furniture.

Using Reiki

Charging a room or space with Reiki is an excellent way to clear any unwanted energy from the area and raise the vibration. Begin by ensuring that you are a clear vessel yourself. The simplest way is to give yourself a quick blast of Reiki, or to draw the Reiki symbols in the air in front of you and walk into them.

The most basic technique for charging a room with Reiki energy is to visualize Reiki symbols, three times each, first on the ceiling, then the floor and then on all four walls, repeating the names of the symbols as you draw them.

Check to see if the room feels different, and repeat if necessary.

If you are not able to draw the symbols physically, do so with your intent and silently chant the names as you visualize the symbols.
You can also Reiki small stones or crystals and place them in the corners of a room to add extra energy.

Welcoming the Ancestors

Many traditions, especially shamanic ones, will welcome the ancestors and invite them to assist with the transition process. If your friend is hoping that particular deceased loved ones will help, such as parents and grandparents, call them by name and welcome them. Place a symbol of them (this could be a photograph or a small item such as a stone or a feather, or a piece of jewellery that belonged to them) on your table or altar.

Many people call the ancestors, spirit helpers and guides with a sacred song as an invocation. Ask for their help, love and guidance in gratitude for the sacred work that will begin. Ask that what occurs be for the highest good of your friend and all life everywhere.

To Finish

Finish the space clearing with a short prayer of intention, such as:

> *'I trust this area is now clear of any negative energy and that it will now remain a place of balance, comfort and love.'*

Light a candle to seal your intention.

In *feng shui* it is common to place a bowl of salt in the middle of a cleansed room, or place small bowls of salt in each corner to absorb any residual negative energy.

4. Personalizing the Space

There are a number of items that you can add to a space to make it sacred for your friend:

- mementos – any personal items that are meaningful to your friend

- talismans such as stones, crystals, prayers, photographs, symbols of peace and hope

- photographs of loved ones

- postcards, pictures, posters and photographs of significant places

- ceramic figurines, spiritual statues, symbols of protective energies

- stones and shells that hold memories of special places

- colour (soft throws, scarves, hangings and quilts)

- flowers and plants

- soft music.

Setting Up an Altar

Altars can be created very simply. You could cover a small table with beautiful fabric, or make a small display on a tray or a shelf. It is important that your friend can see it and that they connect with its meaning.

Lighting

There should be nothing harsh or jarring in a room when someone is dying. Try not to use bright lights, and wherever possible use candles or nightlights instead. Keep them lit all through the night. A soft, glowing light is kind to dying eyes, and burning candles can also bring feelings of peace and safety.

Keep a torch by your side, though, in case you need more light quickly.

Sound and Music

Hearing is the final sense we lose. Even if someone appears to be deeply asleep, sedated, unconscious or in a coma, they can probably still hear you and understand what you are saying. Always speak kindly and softly to your friend, and tell them what you are doing or who is coming to visit them. If you have to leave the room, let them know that you are leaving, and why.

Be sure to use their own name, rather than 'Mr' or 'Mrs', or 'nan' or 'uncle'. Hearing your own name spoken to you can be very intimate. Our name carries a specific energy, our unique essence, and hearing it brings a sense of belonging.

Also, the spoken word – or chanting, singing and music – touches the auditory nerve and runs across the floor of the skull into the brainstem, from where the auditory impulses are relayed upwards to consciousness or, as the ancients believed, the soul. Thus we have the potential to connect not just to a friend's normal hearing and understanding, but also to their soul hearing.

Encourage visitors and loved ones to avoid difficult and jarring conversations while with the dying friend. However, if visitors are honest and truthful in a gentle, loving way, it can bring great relief to the dying. No one should be afraid to shed tears, but loved ones can reassure the dying person that as much as they are loved, it is OK for them to go when they are ready.

Instruments such as drums or bells are used in many traditions at this time. The sounds of nature can also be very healing.

Prayer

You might like to find some prayers in keeping with the dying person's tradition. These could also include poems, psalms and extracts from spiritual books.

Silence

There is, of course, sometimes no need for words at all – silence can touch the heart and have a profound healing effect. It is also one of the most important aspects of creating a ritual (*see pages 137–140*).

5. Creating a Tranquil Atmosphere

There are numerous things that you can do to create a tranquil atmosphere and make your friend more comfortable:

- Ensure the room is clean, fresh and clutter-free.
- Bring the outside in with scented bulbs and blossoms, garden flowers, orchids, stones and shells.

- If possible, make sure there is a good view of the outside world from the bed.

- Change the sheets frequently – at least every other day. The bed linen can be washed with rose or lavender water.

- Add colour and comfort with lovely cushions, soft fabrics, photos and pictures.

- Provide a CD player, radio or iPod (with headphones) and a selection of CDs and talking books; also a laptop and a torch.

- Spritz the air with essential oils or scented floral waters (*see pages 117–121 and 123–124*).

- Provide soft lighting or candles for quiet times.

- Make sure scented soaps and hand creams are available.

PERSONALIZING A ROOM

The room should reflect the very essence of the dying person and should be an uplifting reminder of happy times, hobbies, holidays and moments shared with loved ones.

Here are some ideas that could both occupy your friend and provide topics for conversations with loved ones and visitors:

- A large jigsaw puzzle

- An album of family photos

- An informal picture book with old and new photos interspersed with written memories and experiences. Encourage friends and family to add to it, especially if they can write about how the dying person has positively shaped or inspired their lives.

- Poetry, cards and drawings from friends and family who live too far away to visit.

- A beautiful bowl filled with slips of paper from friends and family, each containing a loving message like, 'Thanks for how loved you always made me feel' or 'Thanks for all those wonderful cakes you made us.' Your friend can chose a slip or two if they are in need of comfort.

Above all, remind loved ones that it's about presence, not presents – time spent with the dying person is worth so much more than flowers and cards.

HELPING CARERS

During this time Soul Midwives can develop strong relationships with carers and provide them with invaluable support.

If you are visiting a friend who is dying at home, try to take some time out to check on the carer. It is all too easy for them to neglect their own needs, or be reluctant to ask for additional help. Remind them to be kind to themselves and encourage them to find time to:

- relax (suggest listening to music, an aromatic bath, walks or exercise in the fresh air, dinner out with close friends)

- nourish themselves (it is easy for carers to forget to eat properly). Encourage visitors to bring nourishing snacks and salads (and cakes!) for the caregiver.

- set limits and request time out when things are becoming too much

- be willing to ask for – and receive – help and support

- find humour and joy in moments shared with the friend and in the kindness of others. Tell them not to feel guilty for finding something funny and having a laugh.

EXERCISE **Caring for Carers**

Carers need support too. Opening questions you could use to offer your support include:

- 'How are you doing? Do you fancy a quick chat?'

- 'Would you like to go out for an hour or two? I could stay here while you are away.'

- 'Who has offered to help you? Do you want me to work with them to coordinate our efforts?'

- 'Would you like me to walk the dog/answer the phone/go to the chemist/do some grocery shopping/watch the children for you?'

Of course, in order to fully support both carer and friend, it is essential to have a detailed knowledge of the dying process. We will look at that next.

SUMMARY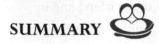

- Advanced Soul Midwives are skilled energy technicians as death approaches.

- They may work with friends on a deep energetic level and non-physical level (the lightbody). They will work within a sacred space and create a 'field' in order to enter a deeper state. This field carries the vibration of unconditional love.

- Sound, essential oils, prayer and silence will all help to create the best environment for the friend.

- Soul Midwives will also attend to practicalities at this time, such as creating a tranquil atmosphere and supporting other carers and family members.

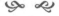

CHAPTER 7

THE DYING PROCESS

'In seeking wisdom, the first stage is silence, the second listening, the
third remembrance, the fourth practicing, the fifth teaching.
KABBALIST SOLOMON GABIROL, C.AD1045

The same process happens with all forms of death. The first stages are
the withdrawal of the elements.

THE WITHDRAWAL OF THE ELEMENTS

The first element to withdraw is Earth, followed by Water, Fire and
then Air. Each elemental stage is also characterized by archetypal
experiences. These manifest in symbolic dreams, conversations and
subtle sensations, and are cross-cultural, because they relate to the
universal human psyche.

   With suicide and assisted suicide, the four elements will withdraw
in the same way, though the separation of spirit and soul (*see pages
60–61*) may be delayed. Many Soul Midwives use psychopomp and soul
rescue work to help souls who have committed suicide.

When people are disconnected from life-support machines, they will almost always have energetically vacated the body. If the decision to leave the body has been taken at soul level, the final phase of soul and spirit separation will still occur.

In a clinical trial in 2001, Dr Pim van Lommel, a cardiologist from the Netherlands, studied a group of patients who had suffered a cardiac arrest and been successfully revived. It is interesting to note that he and his research team found that 62 of the patients (18 per cent) had had a near-death experience and of these 41 (12 per cent) had described a core experience in keeping with the withdrawal of the elements.

The four stages of dying in order of withdrawal of the elements:

Earth

The Earth element is linked to the skeleton, flesh and bones. The withdrawal of this element can be a long, gradual and hardly perceptible process which may last as long as eight to ten years.

Earth is related to our strength and vitality – our zest for life. At the beginning, the Earth withdrawal phase manifests as tiredness and lack of energy. At the end, it presents as frailty, weakness and all the other obvious signs of old age.

Physical Signs

The Earth withdrawal is characterized by a great weariness and lack of sparkle. Friends may sit for long periods in a chair and find simple tasks require more effort. They may begin to lose enthusiasm for activities they used to enjoy. They may complain of aches and pains in their limbs and bones. Their complexion will fade and take on a greyish hue. Their sitting posture will become stiffer. Eventually, they may find it difficult to get out of bed or to sit up at all.

The strength to grasp objects will diminish, and friends may find it hard to keep a firm grip on objects such as cutlery (an indicator of full Earth stage). They often ask for extra pillows, and for bedclothes to be removed because these feel too heavy against the skin. They feel drowsy and find it harder and harder to open their eyes.

It is as if the body is sinking under the earth, becoming smaller and weaker. There may even be a sinking feeling, as if falling, going underground or being crushed by a great weight.

Sense Affected

The Earth element affects the sense of smell. A friend may be repelled by certain familiar smells, but yearn for others. Their own personal smell may also change: there may be a mustiness or tang to the skin. It is almost an autumnal odour. The Soul Midwife may also notice a change of smell in their breath or excretions.

Emotional Signs

Friends may become needy and tearful, and often don't like to be left alone for too long. They may express a fear of the dark or long periods of silence. There is a sense that they feel deep loneliness and isolation and are unable to connect with others.

Dreams and Sensations

Dreams at this stage are often characterized by fearful images, dark holes, chasms and cliff edges. A friend may drift between states of agitation and drowsiness and may mention dreams of shimmering mirages.

Water

The Water element relates to blood, taste and liquids.

People can slip between the Earth and Water stages and flip between the two.

Physical Signs

There may be difficulty in moving the tongue, chewing and swallowing. The tongue may feel rough. The teeth may hurt and the gums ache. Chewing can bring on a headache and fatigue.

Other signs include losing control of bodily liquids, for example, the nose runs, the eyes water and there may be dribbling from the corner of the mouth; there may also be incontinence or seepage from immobile limbs.

Cognitive hearing loss also occurs; it is as if the friend is no longer quite able to process what you are saying. It is almost as if they are beginning to form a cocoon around themselves.

Sense Affected

The Water element affects the sense of taste. The friend may complain that food and drink taste strangely different, perhaps sweeter or more acidic, or dryer and rougher to the tongue. They may request specific food, such as boiled eggs, liver, or paté on toast, and then feel nauseous when it arrives. They may enjoy soup and fresh fruit smoothies, however.

Emotional Signs

The friend may mention that they feel lonely, and demand more attention. Even if they have been feisty and strongly independent in the past, they may suddenly become fragile, weepy and clingy. They may begin to reminisce, particularly about their mothers. Soul wounds may manifest during this stage, when emotions and deep-seated issues are rising to the surface.

Dreams and Sensations

There may be a sensation of being pushed through water, or floating on it, or sinking and drowning in it. The friend may feel overwhelmed and unable to 'get their head above water' or 'stay afloat'. Their dreams may feature swirling wisps of smoke and an undulating haze, walking on water, swimming underwater, paddling through shallow water, drinking water, drinking mystical drinks, becoming waterlogged or having to hold their breath in order to escape to safety by going underwater.

Fire

The Fire element relates to the major organs of the body: heart, lungs, liver and kidneys. It can be quick to withdraw and this stage may only last a couple of days or even hours.

Physical Signs

There may be sudden and dramatic temperature fluctuations, ranging from shivering with cold to burning with fever and wanting to kick off the bedclothes. During the cold phase, the skin will look dry, sallow and parched. In the hot phase, there may be vivid flushing. There may be excessive sweating or no moisture in the skin at all. The lips become cracked. The mouth and nose will dehydrate. The nose may bleed easily and profusely. The person cannot digest food or drink.

There may be itching, scratching, restlessness and agitation. The friend may make plucking motions or appear to be knitting or teasing with their hands.

Eventually, as the Fire stage gives way to the Air stage, the feet and hands will start to feel cold as warmth seeps away from the extremities and towards the heart. You may be able to feel, or even see, a steamy heat rising from the crown chakra.

Sense Affected

The Fire element affects the sense of sight. As it withdraws, the peripheral field of vision narrows and the person is only able to focus on what is straight ahead. For this reason, when you visit, stand at the foot of the bed to introduce yourself before sitting down beside your friend.

As the physical vision decreases, however, the inner vision expands. Friends may talk of seeing dancing lights, colours, loved ones and pets who have already passed on, or angels and religious figures. They often recognize that they are dying and may even tell you when they are going to die.

Emotional Signs

Periods of clarity and confusion will eventually transform into calm, detached acceptance.

Dreams and Sensations

The friend may see shimmering red sparks and feel a sense of panic and urgency. They may appear restless, apprehensive or full of fear and anxiety. They may feel a need to escape and get away from a brooding, menacing presence. Encounters with unknown visitors may occur.

Air

The Air element relates to the lungs and ears.

Physical Signs

The friend will experience a withdrawal and lack of connection. There will be a lack of interest in visitors – a sense of going within. Breathing becomes laboured and erratic. There may be rasping and panting and irregularity between breaths. Some breaths may appear to be missed altogether. The in-breaths may be short and snatched and the out-breaths weaker and longer. The death-rattle may be present. Eyes may roll upwards or be tightly shut. There may be a large bowel evacuation.

Sense Affected

The Air element affects the senses of hearing and touch. The hearing is the last sense to go. Quite often friends hear insistent buzzing noises.

Emotional Signs

Friends may cry out, often in their sleep.

Dreams and Sensations

The friend may experience hallucinations, visions (e.g. flaming torches) and visits from dead relatives or enlightened beings. They may talk of tunnels of light. They may experience an overwhelming sense of love and connection with the universe

Dominant Elements

If your friend is dominant in a particular element, because of their personal characteristics or astrological chart (e.g. born under the 'Water' sign of Scorpio), they will experience the withdrawal of that element with double the intensity. It is worth tuning in to your friend's energy to feel which element is dominant with them. Likewise, you could also ask them their birth/astrological sign to give you an indication of which element they may need extra assistance with in their journey.

Below is a table of astrological signs and their corresponding elements:

Birth sign	Birth dates	Corresponding element
Capricorn	23 December–19 January	Earth
Aquarius	20 January–19 February	Air
Pisces	20 February–21 March	Water
Aries	22 March–20 April	Fire
Taurus	21 April–21 May	Earth
Gemini	22 May–22 June	Air
Cancer	23 June–23 July	Water
Leo	24 July–23 August	Fire
Virgo	24 August–23 September	Earth
Libra	24 September–23 October	Air
Scorpio	24 October–22 November	Water
Sagittarius	23 November–22 December	Fire

THE OPENING OF THE CHAKRAS

There are seven main chakras, or energy centres, in the body, sited between the base of the spine and the top of the head. They store the vital life force described in Eastern medicine as *prana*, *chi* or *ki*. Although they are invisible, they can sometimes be sensed as swirling wheels of coloured energy. When we die, they lose their vitality and start to open wide, starting from the base chakra upwards.

Chakra Correspondences

Here is a list of the chakras and their correspondences:

The Root Chakra

- **Position on the body:** Perineum, base of the spine between anus and genitals
- **Energy location:** Feet, ankles, legs, knees, thighs and large intestine, forming an energetic gateway between us and the Earth
- **Colour:** Red
- **Planet:** Saturn
- **Element:** Earth
- **Yin/Yang:** Masculine/Yang
- **Musical note:** C
- **Sephira:** Malkuth
- **Archangel:** Sandalphon
- **Crystals:** Garnet, haematite, ruby, zircon
- **Incense/oils:** Cedarwood, lavender, myrrh, musk, patchouli

The Sacral Chakra (also called the water chakra)

- **Position on the body:** The sexual organs and upwards towards the navel
- **Energy location:** All fluid functions of the body; ovaries, testes, womb
- **Colour:** Orange
- **Planet:** Pluto
- **Element:** Water
- **Yin/Yang:** Feminine/Yin

- **Musical note:** D
- **Sephira:** Yesod
- **Archangel:** Gabriel
- **Crystals:** Amber, carnelian, red jasper
- **Incense/oils:** Jasmine, rose, sandalwood

The Solar Plexus Chakra

- **Position on the body:** Between the naval and solar plexus centre
- **Energy location:** Pancreas and adrenals
- **Colour:** Yellow
- **Planet:** Mars and the sun
- **Element:** Fire
- **Yin/Yang:** Masculine/Yang
- **Musical note:** E
- **Sephira:** Hod and Netzach
- **Archangels:** Michael and Haniel
- **Crystals:** Amber, citrine, tiger's eye, yellow jasper
- **Incense/oils:** Bergamot, carnation, cinnamon, rose, vetivert, ylang ylang

The Heart Chakra

- **Position on the body:** In the cardiac area, the region of spiritual and physical heart

- **Energy location:** Heart, thymus and immune system

- **Colour:** Emerald green or rose pink

- **Planet:** Venus

- **Element:** Air

- **Yin/Yang:** Feminine/Yin

- **Musical note:** F

- **Sephira:** Tiphareth

- **Archangel:** Raphael

- **Crystals:** Green: chrysophase, emerald, green aventurine, green jade, green tourmaline, malachite, moldavite, peridot; pink: pink tourmaline, rhodochrosite, rose quartz

- **Incense/oils:** Bergamot, melissa, rose

The Throat Chakra

- **Position on the body:** In the throat region at the base of the neck

- **Energy location:** The thyroid gland, lungs, vocal cords, jaw, breath

- **Colour:** Blue

- **Planets:** The moon and Mercury

- **Element:** Aether

- **Yin/Yang:** Masculine/Yang

- **Musical note:** G

- **Sephiroth:** Geburah and Chesed

- **Archangels:** Khamael and Tzadkiel

- **Crystals:** Aquamarine, blue lace agate, blue sapphire, lapis lazuli, turquoise

- **Incense/oils:** Chamomile, myrrh

The Third Eye Chakra

- **Position on the body:** Between and just above the physical eyes

- **Energy location:** Pituitary gland, left eye, base of skull

- **Colour:** Indigo

- **Planets:** Neptune and Jupiter

- **Element:** Water

- **Yin/Yang:** Feminine/Yin

- **Musical note:** A

- **Sephiroth:** Binah and Chokmah

- **Archangels:** Ratziel and Tzaphkiel

- **Crystals:** Amethyst, fluorite, lepidolite

- **Incense/oils:** Geranium, violet

The Crown Chakra

- **Position on the body:** The crown of the head (known as the anterior fontanelle in a newborn child)

- **Energy location:** Right eye, cerebral cortex, pineal gland, upper skull, skin

- **Colours:** Violet, white and gold

- **Planet:** The sun

- **Element:** Fire

- **Yin/Yang:** Masculine/Yang

- **Musical note:** B

- **Sephira:** Kether

- **Archangel:** Metatron

- **Crystals:** Clear quartz, diamond, selenite

- **Incense/oils:** Frankincense, lavender, rosewood

THERAPEUTIC WORK

The key to working with a friend going through these stages is to ensure that the energy keeps flowing. Soul Midwives are able to detect and release blockages which may be hindering the dying process and creating pain and discomfort for the friend.

All the tools we use at this point are energy based, such as sound, oils, soothing touch, vibrational remedies and hands-on or colour healing. For example, some therapists use light torches which focus a beam of coloured light onto an acupressure point or chakra to help clear specific energy blockages.

The focus of our therapeutic work at this stage centres on the physical body of the friend and also the lightbody. Remember that the lightbody is the sum of all the subtle energy bodies put together, including the physical body. Imagine an onion with its rings. Each ring is another layer of energy, and each layer affects all the others.

Although the lightbody is invisible to most people, it can be seen and felt after an attunement and with continued practice. Working with it may take several years of guided practice, however, and is not performed by all Soul Midwives. Dedicated study of vibrational medicine is recommended for this level of work.

Diagnosis

However we choose to work, the key to our diagnostic work is understanding that everything is governed by vibration. Our bodies and souls vibrate within their own individual spectrum of frequencies.

The Aura

The aura is the outer protective energy sheaf around the physical body. It is a three-dimensional energy field that surrounds all matter: people, animals, trees and plants all have auras.

Some people can see auras and describe them in terms of size and colour. In a healthy person, the aura will be oval in shape and extend 2–3 m (8–10 ft) around the physical body.

The aura is made up of two parts: the etheric, which is next to the skin, and the energetic, which extends like a colourful plume around the body for about 40 cm (1½ ft). The two together can tell us how strong the person's energy field is and how it is being affected by their physical health, mental activity and emotional wellbeing.

The etheric aura looks like a thin band of smoky grey film with a misty outline about 2 cm (¾ in) wide. When we are awake, it is compressed and thin, but it expands during sleep and unconsciousness to absorb universal *chi* energy and becomes noticeably softer and fuller.

The energetic aura is much wider than the etheric and can be seen around the body in swirling coloured bands. It has depth and texture, warm and cool areas, and parts of it tingle and dance with flashes of coloured light and streamers.

When people are dying, the auras change as each stage of death is completed:

- The etheric aura begins to fade with old age, or as the dying person becomes weaker. Eventually it becomes almost undetectable. However, a couple of days prior to death it begins a rapid transformation, becoming softer and fuller. This occurs as the chakras open wide and begin to discharge pulsating streams of heightened energy into the aura. This change can be seen by sensitives as a vivid luminous glow.

- The colours of the energetic aura begin to fade during the weeks before death, until there is only a faint glow left, giving the aura a pale and hazy appearance. As with the etheric aura, however, the energetic aura expands just prior to death due to the opening of the chakras. This often has the effect of temporarily revitalizing the dying person.

Observing auras can also be a useful way of gauging how much time a dying person is spending out of their body in preparation for finally leaving. When someone is 'out of body', the aura virtually disappears – it's as if just a pilot light is left burning.

You can teach yourself to see auras, but it is easier to sense them with your hands. First of all, however, it is important to prepare yourself properly.

Preparing Yourself

Before doing any kind of energy work with a friend, take the time to prepare yourself:

- Before you meet your friend, you must ensure that you are physically grounded. Have you eaten? Are you hydrated? Are you clean and presentable? Are you feeling healthy and robust?

- Are you mentally prepared? Have you left your day-to-day worries and concerns behind at home? Are you able to greet your friend with a light heart and a smiling face?

- Are you energetically prepared? Preparing yourself energetically is a very personal thing. It is a good idea to create a ritual for yourself before you work with a friend: a simple prayer or mantra, a moment spent linking with your guides, a short personal healing session and a quick ritual/visualization of protection. Use whatever works for you, but make sure that you take the time to sit quietly and ground yourself before you meet your friend. You might like to try the following exercise:

EXERCISE **Attuning Yourself**

- Empty your mind and focus on the Soul Midwifery work you are about to begin

- Take 10–15 deep breaths to concentrate on checking your body to clear it of any aches/pains or distractions (such as hunger, worry about what shopping you need to get, etc.)

- Then ground yourself by imagining yourself sending roots down into the earth.

- Place your hands on your friend's foot, or hold their hand, and try to feel their energy field. This takes some practice, but the more you do it, the easier it is to pick up the energy/mood/feelings of the person with whom you are going to start working.

- Once you feel in resonance with them (this may feel as if you are subtly merging with them), protect yourself in a bubble of light and open your heart. As you open your heart and concentrate on working with love, your aura will automatically expand.

- Power up by inhaling deeply and breathing energy and strength into your own body. Do this until you feel strong and clear.

- Set the intention to assist your friend in any way that aligns with their highest self and is for their highest good.

- When this seems to have happened (you will feel it because everything will be in alignment), you can begin.

Fortunately, in this kind of work there is a built-in safety valve from the universe: we will only be given the power that we can safely and responsibly use. Anyone who goes beyond their limits will find their gift evaporating.

EXERCISE **Examining a Friend to Assess their Field**

Before you begin your healing work, you must double-check that you are in balance and fully protected.

- Greet your friend at the foot of the bed, explaining who you are and why you have come.

- Tune into your friend by holding their feet and picking up their vibration.

- Then, slowly working up and down the body, with your hands 1.5–2 cm (4–5 in) above them, tune into their hearts and sense what they are experiencing. Begin to feel their vibration. You will need to be able to clearly recognize your own vibration in order to define where your energy field meets that of your friend. Failing to do this will confuse your ability to intuit how they are feeling and where they may be blocked.

- Sense which element is naturally dominant with your friend, and consider which elemental stage of withdrawal they are engaging in at this time. If you are able to see the lightbody, you will also be able to scan the etheric, astral, emotional, mental and causal bodies to look for anomalies.

- Then begin to scan your friend's physical body for blockages. These will be areas of a different quality – perhaps hot or cold, prickly, dense or woolly.

- If you need confirmation, scan the aura using tingshas or an energy chime bar or singing bowl. You will hear the tone dip where there is a blockage.

- Hovering above the blockage with the note toning will often be enough in itself to release the stagnant energy. You can also use your hands, or breath, to clear the blockage.

Once the flow of energy has been restored in the lightbody, the friend usually feels much calmer and steadier.

Therapeutic Techniques

Complementary therapies are the 'bread and butter' work of a Soul Midwife. Below are those which are most commonly used, but there are many other energy healing disciplines which can be adapted and used with the dying.

Although the friend's illness has manifested on the physical level, always try to look *behind* the symptoms when you are working.

Please check the regulations in your country for safe practice and insurance purposes. After that, use your hands, your heart and your experience and you can't go wrong.

Aromatherapy

Nothing stimulates the senses more quickly than the power and essence of smell. Essential oils work on body and mind, encouraging healing at a subtle level as well as encouraging a positive outlook. Used regularly, oils promote calm and tranquillity and most people really enjoy them.

Essential oils can be used in many ways with the dying, but if you are not a trained aromatherapist, do not embark too lightly on treatments with them. Properly used, they are very safe indeed, but some oils present hazards and even small amounts of oil can build up to a toxic level in the body over a period of time.

Aromatherapists always dilute essential oils with a base or carrier oil for use on the skin (in the proportion 3 per cent essential oil to carrier oil). Therapists usually use sweet almond or grapeseed oils, but peach kernel, apricot kernel and particularly avocado oil are all rich and nourishing for dry and ageing skins. Consequently, carrier oils are good products to use in conjunction with a gentle foot or hand massage. Bear in mind nut allergies when choosing carrier oils.

If you are using oils in conjunction with a hand or foot massage, the massage must be very gentle, and you must always avoid areas around tumour sites. Also, please note some oils should not be used with friends with certain conditions.

OILS TO AVOID WITH THE DYING

The following essential oils should be avoided when friends are suffering from:

- *Cancer:* Anise (aniseed), basil, fennel and nutmeg

- *Oestrogen-dependent cancers:* Anise (aniseed), bergamot, citronella, eucalyptus, fennel, lemongrass and melissa

- *Heart disease:* Peppermint (the energy signature is too strong)

- *Kidney disease:* Bay, cinnamon and clove

- *Liver disease:* Anise (aniseed), basil, bay, cinnamon and clove

---

Always check an authoritative guide to aromatherapy (*see Recommended Reading*) before using an oil on a friend.

Oils For Use With the Dying

Many essential oils have intense antiseptic qualities which are far stronger than some of their commercial equivalents. Lavender, lemon and thyme are particularly known for this and can be extremely useful in the sick room, where they can be used in burners or diluted with water in a spray to clear and sweeten a room.

The following oils will ease fear:

- bergamot
- chamomile
- frankincense
- geranium

- lavender

- marjoram

- neroli

- sandalwood

The following oils can bring a sense of balance and equilibrium, particularly as your friend journeys from one elemental stage to another:

- cypress

- elemi

- fennel

- peppermint

- ylang ylang

The following oils are particularly good for use with the dying:

- **Calendula:** A soothing and gentle oil with a light energy signature.

- **Elemi:** Its name is derived from the Arabic phrase meaning 'as above, so below', and this tells us something of the oil's effect on the emotional and spiritual planes. Elemi oil brings mind, body and spirit in alignment with each other. It is a great oil to burn in a diffuser (*see below*), as it induces deep calm without drowsiness – good for visiting loved ones too!

- **Fragonia:** This has become the oil of choice in Soul Midwifery because it works very quickly to restore balance when the elements are withdrawing and energy shifting.

- **Frankincense:** This oil sets the spirit free. It has the ability to slow down and deepen the breath and hence bring calm. It is useful in helping people break links with the past, expand their consciousness and heal old wounds. It also assists inward reflection.

- **Geranium:** Warm, nurturing and loving, this oil balances highs and lows. In times of uncertainty it helps prevent excessive sensitivity.

- **Helichrysum:** Useful for spirit release; like the sun, this works with the finer aspects of spirit energy.

- **Kewra:** This is a very expensive oil, and hard to source, but very useful. It is good for manifesting a deep soul connection.

- **Lavender:** While this oil is calming and soothing, its real strength is in restoring balance, which makes it invaluable when someone is dying. It is also great for muscular pain and insomnia. Warm aromatic baths with lavender can help a friend in the early stages of an illness.

- **Myrrh:** This oil promotes a deep connection to spirit. It helps with endurance and strength and promotes inner silence.

- **Palo santo:** A powerful shamanic oil that is good for releasing negative energy.

- **Petitgrain:** A good sedative oil and antidepressant with a wonderfully fresh and flowery aroma, petitgrain is comforting in convalescence and can help anyone who is run down.

- **Ravensara:** Useful for releasing secrets and karmic contracts. Ravensara is a relative newcomer to Soul Midwifery, and I am still researching its properties, but it has had very profound effects on friends who have been troubled by karmic phobias and soul burdens.

- **Rose:** Great for soul wounds (particularly for women), broken hearts, grief, jealousy and anxiety.

- **Rosewood:** This oil brings balance, eases the mind and helps connect loved ones and carers. It is good for stress and can stabilize energy levels and restless minds.

- **Sandalwood:** A traditional transition oil, this is earthy, safe and effective, and stabilizes mind, body and spirit. Sandalwood also promotes courage and alleviates loneliness and obsession.

- **Spikenard:** This is the ancient and sacred oil used by Mary Magdalene to anoint Jesus on the night of the Last Supper. It was used to strengthen his energy field. It was very effective (and costly) 2,000 years ago, but is now slightly underpowered for the average human energy signature. However, it still has its place in transition work. It is very good for anyone who is anxious and tense and, like frankincense, it helps people let go of old pain and emotional blocks, so it is useful when working with soul wounds. It is not suitable for everyone, as it can trigger past-life flashbacks, but it is helpful for the transition of priestly archetypes. It has an unusual smell which many people find repulsive, so it is worth mixing it with other oils such as geranium, lavender, mandarin and rose.

EXERCISE Lifting the Energy of a Room

One of the simplest ways to use essential oils is to put them into an electric diffuser to lift the energy of a room.

Choose an essential oil or oil blend based on the friend's particular needs.

Start with just one or two drops and increase if necessary once you have gauged how the friend tolerates the aroma.

Tiger balm or peppermint help reduce the effects of sick room odours. Peppermint oil is particularly useful. If you place gauze in the top of the bottle with the lid off, it works as an air deodorizer. It is a much more pleasant air freshener than most commercial air deodorizers. You can also apply peppermint oil to a face flannel and place it near a fan.

(*See also Hydrolats opposite*.)

Colour Therapy

Colour, like smell, can have a great influence on our moods and emotions. When used therapeutically, it can enhance the effects of other forms of healing. Some colours will soothe, some will stimulate, others will inspire. The colours we choose when we are working with the dying can have a profound effect.

Soul Midwives often drape coloured silk squares on parts of the body to bring a sense of calm and security during treatments:

- **Red:** encourages adrenaline and can be used to stimulate empowerment, positivity and focus in the early active stages of an illness

- **Orange:** an appetite-stimulant; friendly and outgoing

- **Yellow:** a very cheerful and sociable colour, useful for alleviating depression

- **Green:** the colour of balance and harmony; relaxing and connecting with nature

- **Pink:** feminine; the colour of heart energy, love, nurturing and softness

- **Blue:** peaceful, calming, stabilizing, balancing and comforting, blue has been shown to reduce blood pressure and respiration and heart rate

- **Purple:** the highest frequency in the colour spectrum, it connects people with their spirituality

- **White:** clean, simple and crisp, yet too sterile for some; a very good background for other colours.

Hydrolats

Hydrolats or hydrosols, also known as flower or floral waters, are the leftover waters from essential oil distillation processes. They are gentler than pure essential oils and are ideal to use with frail friends who may not be able to tolerate the more powerful oils.

Because they are water based (with an affinity to the Water phase of the dying process) and more delicate than many of the pure concentrated oils, they are also perfect for working with the elderly or young children.

You could consider using the following:

- **Angelica root:** thought to provide strength to women

- **Atlas cedar:** grounding and calming and combats negativity

- **Bulgarian rosewater:** ideal for refreshing parched skin

- **Clary sage:** good for stress

- **Lemon verbena:** a powerful relaxant and sedative, but do not use on the skin

- **Orange blossom:** acts as an antidepressant, relaxes the body and uplifts the spirit

- **Sandalwood:** deeply grounding, and useful with colour and chakra work; calming; can alleviate depression and bring inner peace
- **Spikenard:** a sedative that can be used for blessings and protection.

Plant Tinctures

Tinctures are probably the most quick and efficient way a friend can benefit from herbs and are especially useful for working with soul wounds. Always buy them ready prepared unless you are a skilled herbalist.

Remember, we never give our friends any tinctures or medicines by mouth. Instead we use the liquid to bathe the aura. This is important, as herbs may react with the medication the friends are taking.

Consider using the following:

- **Red clover:** As a plant essence tincture, red clover helps us individuate and release our psychic ties to the community. This is also a great emergency mixture when assisting ungrounded souls or traumatized friends or family members.
- **Red penstemon or lion's breath:** This tincture has the capacity to free a friend from personal limitations by promoting soul courage. It transforms negative beliefs about ability and endurance in the face of adversity.

Reiki

The word *Reiki* means 'universal life-force energy' and the practice is a powerful form of touch healing originating from Japan. Reiki energy goes wherever the healing is needed and works on the physical, emotional, mental and spiritual levels simultaneously.

If you are already a Reiki practitioner, go use those hands! The Reiki symbols can be very useful in releasing energy blocks (Cho-Ku-Rei), releasing soul wounds (Sei-He-Ki) and even karmic issues (Hon-Sha-Ze-Sho-Nen). You may also find that when someone is dying and their energy signatures begin to transform, they become much more receptive to the healing energy – almost like a child or animal. Consequently, they may readily absorb the energy and only require short healing sessions.

If you have not worked with Reiki before, find a local practitioner and have a Reiki healing yourself. It is much easier to understand the concept of energy healing if you have experienced it.

Soothing Touch

Also known as Therapeutic Touch, Jam Che or Gentle Touch, this may involve Reiki, Gentle Touch or hands-on healing. It will always be given as the friend lies down in bed, fully clothed. A session of 30 minutes or so is usually sufficient.

Sound Baths

Sound baths are a wonderful offering at the bedside. They are a massage with sound, which is usually created with percussive instruments – singing bowls, finger cymbals, chimes, rain sticks and crystal sound bowls, but also harps and sounding bowls.

Talismans

Many people like to have a talisman with them – a significant religious item, an angel ornament, a ring, a crystal or stone, etc., that brings a feeling of protection. If your friend does not have one, you could always give them a cleansed rose quartz tumble stone to hold. It's even better if it's in the shape of a heart. You can also 'power up' stones with Reiki or simply your loving intent.

Ceremonies and Rituals

We all deserve to die in peace. Simple bedside end-of-life rituals may help a person release anxiety about death and also see their present situation in a new light. Traditional ceremonies such as anointing may prepare someone for death and facilitate forgiveness.

Anointing

Anointing is a sacred act of deep service. It may be very effective when the dying person reaches the Water stage. Traditionally it was seen as a cherishing act to prepare and nourish a soul (both physically and spiritually) before a sacred journey. The power of the intent used before anointing is what gives the act its healing quality.

EXERCISE **Preparing for and anointing your friend**

Prepare yourself by meditating and clearing your mind before you begin.

You will need:

- a bowl of water

- a few drops of either amber or sandalwood essential oil

- a small amount of pure oil base such as almond oil (unless the friend has a nut allergy) or an unscented massage oil, or organic argan oil, avocado oil, cold-pressed passionfruit, rose macerate, sea buckthorn or St John's wort macerate.

If you are confident with essential oils, you might consider substituting the following for the amber or sandalwood oil:

- Angelica is good for clear, purposeful transition. It is pure and strong. It is the oil of choice for friends seeking awareness at transition.

- Ravensara/rose oil (mixed) can help release deeply held anxieties and soul burdens.

- Rosemary is ideal for a young soul who is resistant to surrendering to transition. It also has an affinity with the afterlife, and with faithfulness between soul mates and twin souls. It is useful, too, when working with a friend's ancestral lines.

- Spikenard can be used for old soul/ priestly/holy woman/ man archetypes.

Focus on what you are going to do, and prepare everything so that the actual anointing is the last gesture you perform.

Set your Intent

Determine the reason *why* you are anointing your friend. As an example, make a statement such as 'I am helping to clear away any obstacles that may be hampering a tranquil and peaceful release.'

Remember to honour the life and energy of the person you are about to anoint.

Purify Yourself

As the anointer, you must first symbolically purify yourself. Dip either hand into the bowl of water and then touch the top of your head, your heart, your left and right palm and your left and right foot. There is no specific order in which to do this as long as each area of your body has been symbolically purified.

Express Gratitude

Gratitude is a sign of letting go. When you are able to be grateful for something that has caused difficulty and pain in your life, it shows that you have moved beyond the surface and into the larger picture: you have grown as a result of the experience. This lets you and the universe know that you no longer 'need' whatever it is in your life for growth. As you prepare to anoint your friend, set the intention that both of you will show gratitude in this way.

The Anointing

When you are ready to anoint your friend, press a small amount of the oil mixture into the crown chakra with your thumb. Follow the same method with the heart chakra and then the feet, just where the toes meet the foot. This is an energetically important area that has strong energy reflexes.

When you have anointed your friend, remember to honour the experience of partaking in this blessing.

(For more on ceremonies and rituals with a friend, see pages 137–140.)

THERAPIES FOR THE WITHDRAWAL OF THE ELEMENTS

As the elements withdraw, certain therapies can be particularly useful in keeping the energy moving and making the dying process as smooth as possible.

Elemental Correspondences

Knowledge of the elements' correspondences with the seasons, diseases, chakras, herbs, oils, archetypes, music and colour can help us to support our friends through the process of elemental withdrawal.

Earth

Animals: Diggers in the earth (e.g. badgers, rabbits); forest dwellers; hoofed animals; insects in the earth (e.g. ants)

Chakra: Root

Colours: Brown and green

Cycle of life: Old age

Direction: North (northern hemisphere); south (southern hemisphere)

Diseases: Arthritis, bone cancer, bowel disease, rectal disease

Dreams: Shimmering mirages, heat haze

Emotional signs of withdrawal: Losing appetite for life

Gender: Feminine

Physical signs of withdrawal: Fatigue, fragility, greyish complexion, weakness

Represents: Body, matter, solidity and Planet Earth

Season: Winter

Sense affected when dying: Smell

Spiritual signs of withdrawal: Questioning long-held beliefs

Symbols: Caves, clay, fields, rocks, salt, soil

Time: Night

Water

Animals: Mythic water creatures (e.g. mermaids, water dragons); sea/water birds; sea creatures; water animals

Chakra: Sacral

Colour: Blue

Cycle of life: Maturity

Direction: West

Diseases: Depression, leukaemia, lymphoma, oedema, pneumonia

Dreams: Walking on water, swimming underwater, wisps of smoke or undulating haze

Emotional signs of withdrawal: Becoming emotional; reviewing relationships, family trauma and personal trauma; revisiting the past

Gender: Feminine

Physical signs of withdrawal: Lips, skin and eyes become parched; loss of control over bodily fluids (incontinence)

Represents: Dreams and visions, love and emotions, mystery

Season: Autumn

Sense affected when dying: Taste

Spiritual signs of withdrawal: Soul wounds surface to be healed

Symbols: Cups, fog, lakes, oceans, rain, rivers, shells, springs, wells

Time: Dusk

Fire

Animals: Cats (all types); desert dwellers (e.g. lizards, scorpions, snakes); mythic fire creatures (e.g. fire dragons, phoenixes)

Chakra: Solar plexus

Colours: Gold, orange, red

Cycle of life: Youth

Direction: North (southern hemisphere); south (northern hemisphere)

Diseases: Appendicitis, gall bladder problems, heart attack, pancreatitis

Dreams: Fire, shimmering red sparks

Emotional signs of withdrawal: Agitation, anxiety, instability, no interest in conversation, preoccupation, restlessness, short attention span, tetchiness

Gender: Masculine

Physical signs of withdrawal: Burning fever and flushes, then chills; tunnel vision

Represents: Energy, passion, the sun

Season: Summer

Sense affected when dying: Sight

Spiritual signs of withdrawal: Clairvoyance, dark night of the soul, prophetic insights/visions, super-sensitivity

Symbols: Flames, heat, heated objects (stones in particular), lava, lightning, rainbow, stars, the sun, volcanoes

Time: Noon

Air

Animals: Birds (eagles, ravens, etc.) and winged insects (butterflies, dragonflies, etc.)

Chakras: Heart, throat

Colour: Yellow

Cycle of life: Infancy and the wonder of childhood

Direction: East

Diseases: Alzheimer's disease, asthma, brain tumours, emphysema and other lung disease

Dreams: Flaming torches and tunnels of light

Emotional signs of withdrawal: Confusion, detachment, distance, forgetfulness, withdrawal into a cocoon

Gender: Masculine

Physical signs of withdrawal: Altered breathing, detachment, drifting in and out of consciousness, sleeping more

Represents: Inspiration, new beginnings, sunrise

Season: Spring

Sense affected when dying: Hearing and touch

Spiritual signs of withdrawal: Having visions and out of body experiences, seeing guides and a bright light

Symbols: Breath, breezes, clouds, feathers, flowers, herbs, plants, smoke, sky, trees, vibrations, wind

Time: Dawn

(Please note that the colours and directions are different in Native American teachings.)

Earth Withdrawal

Oils: cedar, geranium, patchouli and sandalwood have an affinity with the Earth stage and will help to bring balance. They may be added to a base oil and used to massage hands or feet, or used in an atomizer or electric diffuser.

Soothing touch: this may also be beneficial now.

Sound work: offering a sound bath, or just sitting and singing lullaby-type songs, or working with a single singing bowl, will encourage relaxation. Muffled drums are recommended at the Earth stage.

Water Withdrawal

Anointing: with water (such as holy water), essential oils or hydrolats mixed in water can be very beneficial (*see page 123*).

Aura Cleanse: homoeopathic or herbal tinctures may be used. Do not use them orally, but in diffusers or as an aura cleanse (rub your hands with the tincture and smooth the aura of your friend).

Oils: recommended oils/hydrolats for this stage are angelica, fragonia, geranium, kewra, orange and rose (*use as described for Earth above*).

Sound work: sound baths with singing bowls and toning, or playing an instrument, particularly anything resonant, or a CD can be very relaxing and healing.

General: if the person is anxious, try tucking a big, soft, cuddly teddy into bed with them. Stroking something soft can be very calming. Blankets in grey/blue tones can also help soothe.

Fire Withdrawal

Oils: recommended oils for this stage are fragonia, frankincense, jasmine and myrrh (*use as described for Earth above*).

Soothing touch: if the friend is anxious during this phase, you may find you can soothe them by holding their hand and moving it in slow circular clockwise movements. Keep eye contact with the friend and talk to them gently and quietly. This can break the pattern of agitation if they are plucking at the bedclothes and generally restless. It also works well with dementia patients, who may view everyone as a stranger.

Sound work: singing softly can also be a non-threatening therapy which releases trapped energy and tension. Offer a soothing sound bath or play stringed instruments or CDs, or a single singing bowl.

General: as your friend begins to cool towards the end of this stage, covering them in warm soft blankets can help. Use your intuition as to the colour, but pale mauves work well at this stage.

Air Withdrawal

Breathing techniques: people may experience anxiety with their breathing at this stage and will often describe it as 'shortness of breath', 'tightness in the chest' or a feeling of 'smothering'. Breathing techniques such as mirrored breathing and liquid light breath are invaluable in easing your friend if their breathing is laboured.

EXERCISE Practising breathing techniques

Mirrored Breathing
- Sit quietly with your friend and synchronize your breathing to match theirs. This may take a few minutes of concentration for both of you.

- When you are breathing in time with them, ask them to try to consciously fill up their lungs and take slightly longer, more controlled breaths. Guide them in taking a deep breath in and then exhaling in a smooth flow while you make the sound *aaaaaahhh*.

- Repeat this for a series of ten or twelve exhalations, until their rhythm is stronger and more confident.

Liquid Light Breath

This technique is a healing and visualization which can help people who are close to the end of life. They don't have to participate physically.

- Place your hands above the friend's chest (not touching).

- Ask them to imagine a stream of golden light flowing from your hands into their lungs.

The golden light then forms a channel for the oxygen to flow through and their breathing will become easier.

~~~~~~

Oils: both fragonia and frankincense are useful at this stage.

Sound work: play relaxing music, particularly flutes and other wind instruments. The sounds of birdsong can also be soothing.

General tips for air withdrawal:

- Ensure that the room is cool (but not chilly), and check that the friend's bedclothes aren't too heavy.

- Open a window for fresh air.

- Use a fan to blow air towards the friend's face.

Knowing When to Stop

None of these therapies should last more than 30 minutes or so. 'Less is more' with energy work at the bedside. Only do what is required and is genuinely helpful.

Occasionally a little healing can give someone the energy they need to greet a visitor or make a phone call, but beware of attempting anything on a grander scale 'just because you can'. If you do, you will swing out of balance with the rhythm of the universe and interfere with your friend's journey. Also, eventually, energy cannot be absorbed any more.

A THERAPEUTIC ACTION PLAN

If you have the opportunity to do so, spend quiet time with your friend finding out how best you can help them. Explain the types of therapies available and then, together, draw up a plan.

It takes time to do this, so don't rush it. The plan also needs to be flexible so that you can bring in new options when required.

A SAMPLE THERAPEUTIC ACTION PLAN

As an example, here is the profile of a friend:

Annabelle

Age: 56

Wants to die at home.

Family: Mother (frail, but wants to help and be involved); older sister, Lucy, who lives two hours away (not close relationship)

Physical disease: Heart failure

Spiritual state: Vulnerable/fragile

Root cause: Probably relates to her husband abandoning her after their third child was killed in a car crash 10 years ago.

Soul wound: Abandonment and lack of self-esteem

Constitutional elemental type: Water

Action plan: Suggest working with rose oil, water violet, gentle music. Annabelle likes massage and healing.

One part of your plan may be creating rituals, ceremonies and blessings together.

CREATING RITUALS, CEREMONIES AND BLESSINGS

Sacred blessings and prayers, letting-go rituals, rituals for unresolved issues (such as anger, remorse or sadness) and purification rituals may all help your friend prepare for their final journey.

There is no right or wrong way to create meaningful ceremonies, as long as the intention is rooted in love and compassion. When you are conducting a ritual, however, please be meticulous in your preparations. Be clear in your mind what you are going to do and say, and aware of your motivation for doing so, and make sure you are grounded and fully present. Creating a ritual and sacred ceremony is very profound for both friend and Soul Midwife alike.

Here are some suggestions for wording a ritual or prayer:

- 'I am helping [friend's name] to clear away any obstacles that may be hampering a tranquil and peaceful release.'

- 'I am helping [friend's name] to finally release the trauma they have been holding within them about [name the traumatic event].'

- 'This act of [ceremony] is to honour and bring to the present memory someone that [friend's name] has lost through the end of a relationship or through death.'

- 'We are [performing this ceremony] in order to release any unhelpful promises or vows or relationships made in the past.'

Use your friend's name, because names have a powerful and spiritual resonance of their own.

It is interesting to note that I often feel the love of family and friends who have passed on when I am conducting a blessing at the bedside.

Here are some blessings and prayers you could use, either as they are or as a basis for blessings and prayers of your own:

A Soul Midwife's Prayer for the Bedside

It is time to let go.

You are safe and loved and you are not alone.

Just fall into my arms and sleep.

You don't have to make things happen –

they will happen on their own.

Let me hold you. Just let go, don't resist.

You are doing so well,

like a feather falling from the sky.

Sink back into soft feathered wings.

You are working hard,

delving deep within yourself,

like a chrysalis changing to a butterfly.

Of course you are weary –

change is hard work.

Your body is tired, but don't be frightened,

just love and all will be well.

FELICITY WARNER

Prayer / Blessing for a Friend at the Bedside

May our dear friend [name] be filled with peace and love.

We light this candle to symbolize their bright, bright soul which is eternal.

Gather, family, friends, gather near and be still in the love that is present.

We allow our beautiful friend the time and freedom to take their journey with our love and blessings.

Dear friend, know that you are loved by each and every one of us.

We know you will be received by love itself when the time is perfect for you.

Hear us and know you are loved.

Our souls embrace you where we never knew separation.

With blessings and love,

Amen

ELIZABETH HORNBY

Scottish Soul Midwives' Blessing

Guardian of my soul,

Be my guiding star.

Light my way past every reef and shoal.

Pilot my ship through stormy waters

To the peaceful harbour

On the waveless sea.

ANON

EXERCISE Creating a Ritual

Jason is a 43-year-old father of three. He is dying from leukaemia. His parents were Catholic, but Jason dropped his faith as a young man and has a deep distrust of the Church. However, now that he is dying, he feels a strong need for a blessing that will enable him to be forgiven for mistakes he has made in his life.

When he was 19 he got his girlfriend pregnant and persuaded her to have an abortion. Now that he is the father of three teenagers, he often thinks about the baby he would have had and feels very guilty about the fact that it was aborted. He now feels that all life is sacred and that he committed a very serious sin.

He split up with the girlfriend. Later he heard that she developed a serious drink problem and never had another serious relationship. He has always wondered if it was partly due to him, as she suffered from deep depression after the pregnancy was terminated.

Jason has shared this with his wife, Jane, but now wants to have a blessing to say he is sorry and seek forgiveness.

What ritual could you create for him?

Suggestions:

- find meaningful objects to create an altar beside his bed

- choose suitable music to begin the ceremony

- write a personal blessing

- mix a beautiful anointing oil for the occasion or source some holy water

SUMMARY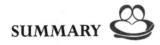

- The dying process involves the withdrawal of the elements Earth, Water, Fire and Air.

- Each element has its own set of correspondences relating to disease, archetypes, seasons, oils, etc.

- Each stage of withdrawal has its own characteristic signs and symptoms affecting the emotional and spiritual aspects of a friend.

- As the elements withdraw, the chakras open in sequence.

- The aura of the dying friend fades.

- The Soul Midwife will use specific oils, tinctures, energy healing techniques and sound to keep the energy flowing at each stage.

- The skill of the Soul Midwife is in keeping the friend comfortable physically, emotionally, spiritually and energetically as the stages progress.

CHAPTER 8

WATCHING WITH THE DYING

'Each human should die with the sight of a loving face.'

MOTHER TERESA

Imagine dying alone and afraid. It is a terrible thought, but sadly, it's a reality for many thousands of people, every day.

Although our dying loved ones usually (but not always) desire us to be with them as they pass away, we, the living, also benefit immeasurably from the experience. The dying are our teachers, and each generation's parting gift is showing us how to go about the journey of dying. They are just a few steps ahead of us in the great scheme of cosmic time, and they are marking the way for when it is our turn.

Thankfully, sitting with a loved one as they pass away isn't an everyday event for most of us. But when we have experienced it, it usually changes our lives forever. Many hundreds of people have shared their most personal stories at my workshops, and the most moving and poignant ones have always been those that have described the precious final hours spent sitting with loved ones.

I never forget these accounts and the love that pours from the remembering and sharing of them. They paint a picture of how people felt as they saw life ebbing away, and what they saw, both in the flesh and in the hollow of their mind's eye. Every poignant detail – the conversations, the expressions on their beloved's face and the tiny inconsequential things that other people said or did – had great significance. You can sense that these experiences have been turning points in the lives of the living.

Revisiting the time when a loved one passed can be a form of self-healing, giving the bereaved the motivation to step back into their lives somehow wiser and more mindful of how precious everything is.

Everyone's death is unique, and the purpose of holding a vigil for the dying is to honour their experience and nurture it by giving them all our attention, kindness and love. Thus the vigil provides a spiritual space for the soul to move peacefully from its physical body.

All around the world, communities have their own traditions for keeping watch over those who are dying:

- In Africa they tell stories about the ancestors so that the dying person can find their way back to them.

- In India they chant holy mantras and anoint the dying one with precious oils.

- In Iceland they sit around a communal fire and gather in the guardian spirits.

- In the western isles of Scotland they mimic the song of the red shank bird to steer the soul home.

- In Tibet they use singing bowls and temple bells to create a growing column of sound energy to envelop the dying one.

Sadly, many of us in the West have forgotten how to keep a vigil. Some people even feel uncomfortable, nervous or 'in the way' if they sit with the dying in a hospital or care home. Many people shy away from visiting the dying altogether, worrying that they won't know what to say, or that they'll feel useless or awkward. But if you bring love with you, it can't go wrong. And being present and bringing compassionate energy into the room is far more valuable than any words. The power of presence is central to all kinds of spiritual practice.

SITTING IN VIGIL

According to Megory Anderson, author of *Sacred Dying* (Marlowe and Company, 2001), 'stillness and silence are the cornerstones of sitting in vigil'.[1] You could also suggest:

- sitting together as a family
- creating a sacred space at the bedside
- keeping focus on the dying person
- remaining calm and centred
- allowing children and pets to participate if they show willingness
- sharing silence
- talking or listening, but above all validating the dying person's experience
- quietly sharing positive memories of being with the dying person
- reading from spiritual texts
- singing, toning, softly repeating mantras or playing inspirational music
- using soothing touch and holding hands
- invoking blessings and fulfilling requested rituals.

For loved ones, viewing the vigil as a sacred ceremony can act as a blessing and allow them to feel something of the eternal. The vigil also creates a peaceful space in which they can begin to make their own transition from carers to mourners. It gives them the time and space to begin to adjust.

So, as well as keeping a vigil yourself, please encourage friends and family to do so too. Sitting in the presence of someone who is dying, and bearing witness, is one of the most devotional acts of loving care we can provide.

Remember that these hours when we sit removed from the daily trivia of life are actually a parting gift from the dying to the living. Soul Midwives sit with many people who have no family or friends, and the experiences we gain are like golden moments.

IS IT TIME?

There are signs that tell us when death is near. You will notice these perhaps two weeks or so before the end, when there is a shift from the pre-active dying phase into the active dying phase.

The Active Dying Phase

The active dying phase is marked by two distinct dynamics: the physical one, as the body begins to shut down and die on a cellular level, and the spiritual one, as consciousness begins to expand and the person starts to spend more time out of their body.

No one can accurately predict how long this final stage will last. The actual letting-go seems to be as much an emotional and spiritual decision as a physical release. Sometimes people rally for a while, wait for someone special to visit, or just withdraw and grow steadily weaker. Drugs can also interfere and mask some of these stages. However, you should notice the following:

Decreasing Sociability

There will be a slow withdrawal from wanting to take part in conversations and activities, which is partly due to increasing physical weakness. This often coincides with a reluctance to get out of bed. The friend may begin to refuse visits from friends and relatives and seek the company of just one or two specific people.

Agitation or Restlessness

The friend may ask to be moved or repositioned often. They may complain that pillows are uncomfortable or that the room is too hot/ cold/noisy/draughty.

Increased Drowsiness and Loss of Consciousness

The friend may sleep for long periods, become muddled and appear to drift in and out of consciousness. They often mumble, reach out for invisible objects, laugh, twitch and make jerking movements.

Unfinished Business

As death approaches, the friend may confide in you about their past and ask for forgiveness. They may wish to see someone to make amends while they still can. If it is not possible to get that person to the bedside, offer to help your friend make a recorded message which you can send on for them.

The Dark Night of the Soul

Jesus appealed to God when he was dying on the cross with heartbreaking vulnerability and rejection, saying, 'My God, my God, why has Thou forsaken me?' His words are often echoed by people experiencing the dark night of the soul. This is the stage when even the most spiritual people temporarily lose their faith and feel utterly abandoned.

This is the very lowest point in the pre-death stage, and it can last for days. It seems to be linked to making a final act of surrender; making the decision to let go and trust in whatever might be. It is often experienced in a much deeper way in people who have very strong religious or spiritual beliefs, and it seems to especially affect priests, nuns, celebrants and healers. It is as if, for a defined period near the point of death, the dying person must detach from all comforting belief systems and their direct connection with the divine. It is an utterly desolate experience.

As Soul Midwives, we can really lend our strength to someone going through this stage. It is helpful to know that it is just another part of the process – another sign that the ego is dissolving. When the dying friend finally emerges from the dark night of the soul and their energy shifts from fear to enlightenment, it can feel like the sun appearing from behind the clouds.

The Physical Signs of Approaching Death

All these signs will alert you that death is approaching. They will be happening at the same time as the physical signs that death is on its way:

Appetite Diminishes

Refusing food at this stage is quite usual, as the body becomes less able to digest it. This can be distressing for carers, so please reassure them that this is normal. Suggest that they offer little treats, such as a spoonful of mashed strawberries and cream or a homemade fruit lolly, but that they shouldn't be offended if these are refused.

Pineapple juice can refresh the mouth and palate if gently applied with a mouth sponge.

Irregular Breathing

A slow or irregular breathing rate may indicate that a friend is getting close to the end of their life. If they are no longer able to speak, a high respiratory rate may be the only indication that they are in pain or having difficulty breathing. Rapid, shallow and intermittent breathing is normal in the final stages (this is called Cheyne Stokes breathing and frequently happens as people get close to death).

If there are periods of apnoea (when the patient stops breathing briefly), notice whether or not their breathing appears laboured. Are they using abdominal muscles to get air in or just taking shallow breaths from the chest?

Poor Muscle Tone

At the very end of life, most patients are bed bound. However, chart whether they are moving their body independently at all. If they are not moving, are their extremities flaccid or contracted? Are they cachectic (extremely thin and wasted)?

Poor Wound Healing

Wounds and infections may not heal as you would expect them to. There may be persistent swelling, particularly in the arms and legs.

Pulse

As people approach death, the heart rate slows and the pulse becomes fainter. Sometimes finding a pulse is extremely difficult. The carotid pulse in the neck may be the last pulse to be seen and/or felt. If it is either very high or very low, it can give you a clue as to how close to the end of life the person is.

Feeling the pulse is also a good way of making initial physical contact. By holding the friend's hand you can assess if their body is warm. If it is and their pulse is high, check their temperature. Having a fever is uncomfortable and may indicate the Fire withdrawal stage. If they are very warm, you may want to offer a cool damp flannel for the forehead.

Skin

Check for warmth of skin. Not only can this tell you if the friend has a fever, but coolness in the limbs may let you know that they are entering the Air stage and approaching death.

All dying patients are at risk of developing bedsores. A pink area that does not blanch when you press on it is a stage one bedsore. Notify the friend's medical team if you notice this, as it is the first sign of skin breakdown.

Also look for swelling in their limbs and abdomen, which shows that fluid is accumulating due to their organs failing.

Urine and Defecation

A decrease in urine output is a good indication of how close to death a friend may be. If they have a urinary catheter in place, it can be easy to see.

Also, if they are still alert, are they eating or have they lost their appetite? When did they last eat? Have they opened their bowels recently? (Often close to death there is a big evacuation.)

PREPARING FOR A VIGIL

You will sense when it is time to begin the vigil. The friend will have lost interest in their surroundings and begun to sink into their own world. There is often a sense of peace surrounding them, and you can feel them withdrawing from their body.

When you feel it is time to start the vigil, you need to prepare both yourself and the space.

Preparing Yourself

When I am setting out to keep a vigil, I always check that I have emptied my mind and left my own worries behind. As Soul Midwife Peter Bengry advises: 'We need to ensure that we are clean within ourselves to be able to act as a vessel for the healing energy. If we are not, it is as if we are receiving divine energy and then sending it through a rusty bucket to our friends.'

EXERCISE **Preparing for a Vigil**

- Sit quietly and ground yourself. Empty your mind of your daily life and your own worries and concerns.

- If you work with spirit guides, call them in to assist you.

- Then ask to connect with the guides of your dying friend. You will sense the guides working as a team to assist you and your friend.

Preparing Your Kit

The vigil may take some time, so it helps to make yourself as comfortable as you can. A soft chair can make all the difference. Take some warm socks or slippers to wear – they will keep you cosy and muffle the sound when you walk around.

What else might you take with you? Here are some ideas:

- A variety of CDs (include relaxation music, hymns, chants and lullabies)

- A journal for writing notes and reflections

- A folder with poems, quotes and prayers

- A mobile phone – turned to silent

- Blankets (for swaddling your friend)

- A snack

- Water to drink and perhaps a flask of tea

- Anointing oils (ready mixed with base oil)

- An electric oil diffuser

- Incense

- Beeswax candles and candle-holders

- Battery candles if you are working in a room where oxygen is being used

- Beautiful cloths to lay items on and larger ones to cover any remaining clutter in the room

- A lamp for reading

- Fresh flowers

Make the room as quiet and as uncluttered as you can and turn down the lights. Light candles if you are able to (this won't be allowed in a hospital or hospice). Otherwise, a battery lantern is a good alternative. I use a selenium crystal light which sits on a changing coloured light base – it is beautiful. If you are reading poems, blessings, meditations or visualizations to your friend, use a book torch rather than putting the lights on.

Bring some things from home to make the room cosier, maybe blankets or shawls in pretty colours, photos of the dying friend's loved ones and pets, or flowers from their garden. Use some essential oils in a diffuser to freshen and scent the air.

Many people who are drifting in and out of life are soothed by the sounds of nature. CDs with the sounds of the sea, birdsong, bees on a summer's day or streams and rivers are gentle on the ear and can block out the busy sounds of the outside world.

Clearing the Space

Before you begin vigiling, clear the space to ensure that no other influences will encroach on this sacred work. Lifting the vibration of the space around the bedside can be invaluable to both your friend and those sitting in vigil.

Essential Oil Sprays

The following oils can be useful in purifying the air and uplifting the energy of a room when vigiling:

- **Frankincense:** to guide the soul home
- **Geranium:** to calm and cleanse
- **Lavender:** to aid sleep and relaxation

- **Rose:** to soothe and lift the spirit

- **Sandalwood:** to help the spirit fly

HOLDING THE SPACE

By holding the space for your friend, you will have the honour of helping to dissolve their fear. This happens slowly, but in unmistakable ways fear or anger will slowly give way to serenity and acceptance.

Encourage your friend to trust and relax into the process. This is especially difficult with someone who is anxious or in pain, but when the person does surrender it feels as if you are both wrapped in the warm, muffling blanket of love. It's amazing every time it happens, but it's especially sacred the first time.

There are many ways of helping a friend move from fear to serenity. One of the simplest is to work with music.

Music and Vigiling

Music can be used during a vigil to release pent-up feelings such as grief, fear, anxiety and sadness, which may be held both tightly and deeply. When these emotions are released, positive ones can take their place and huge shifts happen.

Some hospitals (mainly in the US) and hospices are providing music at the very end of life, with Soul Midwives and thanatologists (specially trained end-of-life therapists) playing harps, flutes, cellos and singing bowls and using the voice. The aim isn't to provide a bedside concert but to create a sanctuary where the dying person can enter a deep state of relaxation.

I once met the composer Sir John Tavener on a beach near where I live. I had been swimming. He was on the shoreline practising yoga and meditating. I can't remember how it happened now, but we ended up sitting on the wet sand and talking about death, dying and the healing power of Indian Ragas for nearly an hour. It was one of the most extraordinary conversations I have ever had. We discussed the power that music has to transcend life in the hours before death, and he drew my attention to the traditional Hindu song 'Praan Tanse Nikle', which is a musical prayer to Lord Krishna, seeking liberation at the time of death.

In Chinese Buddhist culture, sutras and mantras are chanted at the bedside, often accompanied by a group of musicians. The most widely used sutras are *Amitabha Sutra*, the *Heart Sutra*, the *Diamond Sutra* and the *Earth Treasure Sutra*, and their ethereal rhythm seems to bring universal peace and comfort.

Here are some of my favourite vigiling tracks:

- Eric Whiteacre, *She Ascends*

- Arvo Pärt, *Spiegal im Spiegal*

- Lynn Morrison, *Cave of Gold*

- Carolyn Hillyer, *Wrapping the Bark*

- Eva Cassidy, *Fields of Gold*

- John Lennon, *Imagine*

There is also a wonderful song called 'Bowl of Oranges' by the singer Bright Eyes, with beautiful lyrics which show us that a simple touch and a kind smile can be all that we need to do to make someone feel stronger. (*See Resources for more ideas.*)

Toning

Toning, creating single-syllable sounds, can be very transformative during vigiling. As sound expert Jonathan Goldman explains: 'Toning transmits key vibratory frequencies, not only through the physical resonators of the lungs and vocal cords, but through the entire neural latticework of the body.' It is best offered to friends who are familiar with hearing the voice used therapeutically.

I was called to the hospice where Emma, a young friend, was dying. She was a professional singer with a wide knowledge of spirituality and the healing that toning can bring. Six or so of us formed an impromptu 'threshold' choir and we softly toned around her bed.

The sounds seemed to weave a harmonic web around us with Emma lying in the middle. They spiralled around us, becoming lighter and sweeter as they rose and created an almost visible vortex of sound.

After a while, we could all feel Emma's energy being pulled upwards through her heart, through the spiral of sound, like a plume being drawn to the light. She left her frail, cancer-wracked body and became a luminous column of light. It was one of the most joyous transitions I have ever experienced.

Conversations

If you know the person who is dying, share your stories and memories. This allows them to see how they have touched other people and lets them know that their life has had meaning.

If you do not know the person, reading from a book of poems can help to soothe them.

If they are still able to speak, ask them to tell their stories or explain the important lessons they have learned so they can be passed down to younger family members. This lets them know they are still valued and appreciated. Be spontaneous and speak from a place that is real and alive for you.

Encourage family and friends to say their goodbyes. They can do this at the bedside even if the person is sleeping. It is important that they take the opportunity to give the dying person their love, to remember the happy times and to say sorry for any past grievances. This avoids regrets later.

Conversation-starters for family and friends:

- 'I love you and I will miss you.'

- 'You are a part of my heart and always will be.'

- 'I am feeling such sadness at the thought of your death and yet I know we will never be far apart.'

Ann Freeman was called to sit with a dying man at the care home where she volunteers:

> He was desperately frightened. His legs kicked out and he clutched at my arm and screamed and shivered with fear. He was like a wild animal and wouldn't lie still in bed, even though he was terribly weak.
>
> For three hours I sat with him. I began by softly talking to him and repeating his name to him over and over. Then he trusted me enough to hold his hand, and then I sang and met my eyes with his. I consciously sent him love and kindness, and gradually I felt him shifting... dropping and dropping, and dropping even further into a place of calm and acceptance. Eventually he died, peacefully, all fear gone, with his eyes looking directly at mine.
>
> It was a beautiful passing.

Sometimes people are unconscious when we are called to work with them and it's too late to find out who they are and to ask them how best we can help them. In this instance we have to work with them intuitively.

When people are unconscious and deep inside their inner soul space, you can feel them shapeshifting, becoming fluid and dissolving. In this situation I request guidance on meeting them inside the sacred space to ask how I might be of service.

ASSISTING THE RELEASE

Indigenous communities understand this time so much better than we in the West. They know the importance of assisting the soul's release rather than desperately trying to keep it here for a moment longer. They will also have a method for helping this release, such as storytelling or singing around the fire with the dying person present.

Sadly, we don't have many dying myths of our own these days, but this lovely story was shared by Soul Midwife Theo Hall:

> I was looking after a lady who was dying and finding it extremely hard to let go. All her family had been to see her and given permission for her to go, but she just couldn't.
>
> I knew that she had been very fond of sewing and knitting – her home was filled with exquisite wall hangings and colourful cushions – so I told her a story about finishing her life's work, comparing it with completing a tapestry.
>
> I described a beautiful handwoven cloth, made up of many different colours, shades and hues, that she had been creating throughout her life.
>
> On the loom and in the warp and the weft were the figures of her parents building their first home and planting the garden with many bright flowers and butterflies. Under the apple trees she had woven herself as a little girl playing with a puppy on a blanket of green and blue.

Then she was shown as a young woman growing up, then as a bride with a handsome husband with his arm around her waist. In the distance her baby lay in a pram under the trees, wrapped in the same blue and green blanket. More children filled the tapestry, and pets as well, until all her life, including her illness, leading up to the present moment was shown.

So many chapters of her life were sewn into the picture, but now the tapestry was complete and it was time to turn the cloth over and finish off and knot off all the ends. Then she would come to the final stitch and it would be time to make the final knot.

Before it was all finished and complete, she could take her time to look at each section and see how her life filled the canvas. Overall, it was a huge and glorious reminder of who she was and the story of her life.

After a while, she knew it was time to cut the final thread and tie the last knot. The work – an heirloom – was now finished and ready to be handed over to the next generation of women, who were busy creating their own pictures in paint and clay, wool and fabric, in words and song.

Her job was done. She could put away her scissors and hang her tapestry on the wall. It was time. She saw a light beyond her sewing-room door, and with no fear at all, she walked through. She did not turn back to look at the tapestry and all she was leaving behind, as she knew that her parents and friends would be in the light ready to greet her.

MEDITATION

A meditation for entering the dying period which can be read aloud as a guided visualization for the friend can also be extremely helpful at this time. Here is an example:

You are tired and weary and the journey has been long.

You are anxious about what may happen as the night draws in.

Time is slow, nothing feels quite the same as it once did, and you are moving gently towards a new horizon.

Journeying towards the end of time.

What is the end? What is time?

Where did it begin? Where will it end?

Perhaps you are thinking about the life you have led, the people you have loved, your family, your pets, the homes you have lived in, the landscapes that you know so well: trees, the sky, fields and forests, streams and hills, cities and towns...

Where will you be next?

Someone comes, sits next to you and takes your hand in theirs.

It is soft and cool and calm.

You can feel love pouring through it from their heart to yours.

Now you are not alone. Someone is with you, bringing you strength and peace and a soothing, healing presence.

You are safe.

Soft aromas soothe you and bring colour and light to your heart.

Memories – a summer's day, children laughing, the smell of flowers, a softly flowing green river, a kingfisher flying along its edge...

The wind rustles in the trees high above your head and the sky turns pink and mauve and golden as evening comes.

The air is filled with soft sounds, gentle murmurings, tenderness and loving thoughts.

Hands stroke away your fears. Their warmth and energy melt your worries and smooth away the pain.

Listen: a beautiful tune fills the room – a glorious, sonorous, luminous, harmonious and melodic calling to the soul.

It sweeps and soars – pure and true.

It bathes your body with healing sound like a bath of swirling notes and light.

Let go, let go... stretch wider as the light pours in, lifting you and filling you entirely.

Like a shower of stars, you see the space around you opening up wider and wider and brighter.

Soft pink, iridescent blue, shimmering green and delicate mauve are dancing, merging together and weaving a cloth of silver-gold.

Warm hands begin to wrap you in a soft blanket which holds you tenderly with pure love and grace.

You are held. You are safe.

Time becomes timeless. Soft whispers in your ear tell you that you are so loved in this perfect moment... you have always been loved... you are the purest form of love imaginable.

You came in love, you are returning to love, you are held in the soft and pure light of love.

Your breath becomes weaker...

Just rest, just be peaceful... just be... for this is the extraordinary moment when you are held between heaven and Earth.

Be and be loved... beloved...

You are not alone...

This is also the time to use the creative visualization that you may have worked on during the pre-active phase. For example:

Now you are beginning to walk through the garden, down the path with the roses... Let's stop to smell their beautiful scent before we go any further.

We carry on down the path and towards the fountain. The water is splashing and making rainbows as we walk underneath the crystal drops.

I can see the boat tied up and waiting for you to start your journey across the water...

GIVING PERMISSION FOR SOMEONE TO DIE

Many caregivers who work with the dying talk about a stage, close to the end, where it feels appropriate to give permission to the friend to pass on. This is something that many family members feel an instinctive urge to do when the time is right.

It's about being ready to cut the ties that bind. It often marks the point where there is no possible return. It is time to say, 'We love you. Our hearts are filled with so much love for you. You'll never be forgotten, but it's OK to go now.'

I was sent this beautiful account from Susan Palumbo, a nurse and Soul-Midwife-at-heart in New York. She describes the first time she initiated this particular conversation and gave permission to a patient to cross over... if and when he was ready:

Jack became known to the nursing staff as 'the man in bed 8'. He was an elderly Jewish diabetic, semi-comatose, with a tube feed in his stomach. The story of his life remained unknown to me, but the numbers stamped on his arm told me he'd spent time in a concentration camp.

His wife, Esther, was tall and thin. She wore big hats and neatly fitted suits and the brightest red lipstick. Daily she would demand 'a full report on my husband's progress'. Then she would sit silently next to Jack's bed for close to three hours.

She seemed cold and sterile, so I decided that if she wouldn't reach him, I would. I began talking to him more, but one day, when I gently jostled his shoulder, he looked angry. I realized then that Esther understood him better than I did.

The next time I saw her, I asked softly, 'How are you doing?' We sat together and her fears, memories and hopes cascaded out like torrents in a waterfall.

Later I saw her reach over to stroke Jack's head tenderly. 'I will manage, Jack. It is okay with me, if you want to go.'

But in the weeks that followed, Jack still lingered.

One day I watched a nurse open a window, saying, 'You can go now.'

When I questioned her logic, she threw her arms up, saying, 'Nurses have been doing this forever. It works. Don't ask me why.'

But Jack lay there unaffected.

I had never had 'the talk' with a dying patient before, but I reached for his hand and told him it was his decision.

His irises were darting back and forth and I felt his thready pulse quickening a little. Gosh, I thought, I'm doing this all wrong.

I opened my heart as fully as I knew how, hoping that even if I botched up the words, he would feel that I was giving my heart to him.

'You are worthy, Jack,' I said. 'As God is my witness, in you I see His light looking back.'

With that, Jack gripped my hand firmly. I sensed he was asking something more of me or God, but I didn't know what. 'Father, please help this man,' I prayed. 'I don't know what to say.'

I waited. Nothing happened.

Suddenly, I remembered a biblical verse I'd learned as a hymn. It began with 'Yahweh' and Jack was Jewish, so I hoped it would be enough. I began singing: 'Yahweh is the God of my salvation, I trust in Him and have no fear.'

Jack's eyes opened slightly and he began to weep.

'Thank you,' was all I could manage to say. I kissed his forehead and left the room.

That night I dreamed of him. He was young, about thirty, wearing a suit and standing beside his bed. Light emanated from him, but it was his smile that mesmerized me, and I was surrounded by the purest love. I knew he was showing me that he was home and saying thank you.

I awakened with joy and glanced briefly at the clock: 3.05 a.m.

Next day, the night nurse confirmed it: 'The man in bed 8 was found already expired at 3.10 a.m.'

'Yes,' I replied. 'His name was Jack.'

SUMMARY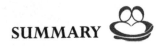

- Prepare yourself for a vigil with an attitude of compassion and love.

- Prepare the space through space clearing.

- Hold the space and listen with your heart as you encourage your friend to move from fear to acceptance.

- Music and toning can help them towards a peaceful release.

- Give permission for someone to die, or encourage their loved ones to do so, if you feel it would be beneficial.

CHAPTER 9

THE SACRED THRESHOLD...
AND BEYOND

'At birth we cry. At death we understand why.'
BULGARIAN PROVERB

When someone is very close to death, they reach a stage when they have a foot in both worlds. The energy that surrounds them is intense and ecstatic. They are reaching the sacred threshold.

The sacred threshold is the boundary separating life from death. Soul Midwives honour it as the place where heaven meets Earth. It is a space where there is no division and no separateness; where all parts of the body, all human beings, all of life and all time zones and parallel universes join together.

All our physical and etheric channels are open as we step across the sacred threshold. All the blockages in the physical and energetic bodies dissolve and our energies are free to flow, enabling our consciousness to expand and merge with the light.

When former Beatle George Harrison died, his wife described how a golden glow filled the entire room – as if it was 'lit by powerful movie lights'. Harrison had followed a spiritual path for many years and had consciously gone towards his death in anticipation of the great enlightenment it might bring.

Author Anita Moorjani also died, but came back to tell of her experiences of crossing the threshold in her book *Dying to Be Me*:

I actually 'crossed over' to another dimension, where I was engulfed in a total feeling of love. I also experienced extreme clarity of why I had the cancer, why I had come into this life in the first place, what role everyone in my family played in my life in the grand scheme of things, and generally how life worked. The clarity and understanding I obtained in this state are almost indescribable. Words seem to limit the experience – I was at a place where I understood how much more there is than what we are able to conceive in our 3-dimensional world. I realized what a gift life was, and that I was surrounded by loving spiritual beings, who were always around me even when I did not know it.

The amount of love I felt was overwhelming, and from this perspective, I knew how powerful I was and saw the amazing possibilities we as humans are capable of achieving during a physical life. I found out that my purpose now would be to live 'heaven on earth' using this new understanding, and also to share this knowledge with other people. However I had the choice of whether to come back into life, or go towards death. I was made to understand that it was not my time, but I always had the choice, and if I chose death, I would not be experiencing a lot of the gifts that the rest of my life still held in store.

THRESHOLD ENERGY

Whether we step across the sacred threshold or step back, threshold energy is extraordinary.

When I first began teaching the energy aspects of Soul Midwifery, the electric charge in the room would build throughout the day until lightbulbs blew, watches stopped and kettles and laptops broke. It was exciting but strange. It was almost as if we had attracted poltergeist activity, yet there was no other evidence of this. What we had done was create an extremely powerful new field.

Waves of high-frequency energy would pulsate around us and these were euphoric times. However, the students returned each morning exhilarated but also completely exhausted. Before we started the day's work, they recounted similar stories of sleepless nights, past-life flashbacks, lucid dreams and visits from deceased loved ones. It was as if the group energy that we had created had the effect of thinning the veils and opening dimensions. The experienced healers and shamanic students in the group quickly understood and enjoyed this, but to those less familiar with energy work, it was very unnerving.

In recent years, there has been a lot of talk about creating fields. To name just a few, there is the 'zero-point field', the 'psi field' relating to psychic phenomena, Ervin Laszlo's 'Akashic field' and the 'morphic field' proposed by Rupert Sheldrake. The common thread between them is that they all describe what happens when there is a similarity between the people experiencing certain phenomena and the phenomena themselves. Just as when two singing bowls of the same pitch are played together, they resonate. This idea of resonance explains how we are able to interact with and expand the energy we are working with at any given time, especially when it's amplified by working as a group.

We create fields in this way every day in ordinary situations, but the resonance created by Soul Midwives working together with the intent and consciousness of love and compassion has enough power in it to have huge effects on physical matter. No wonder a room full of Soul Midwives, or even one or two carrying the frequencies of love and compassion, seems to have such a huge effect on the environment in which they are working. Many people have commented on this.

Biologist Rupert Sheldrake's theory of morphic resonance helps to explain why this is happening. Sheldrake suggests that members of the same species, being 'on the same wavelength', are able to tap into information that pertains uniquely to them. Enormous fields can be involved, such as the collective unconscious of a whole species, or much smaller fields, where members resonate in more focused zones of vibration and create their own 'private frequency'.

Sheldrake also suggests that morphic fields may explain the mechanics of human memory. Instead of memories being stored in the brain, he proposes that they are stored in the morphic field. Our brains retrieve them by tapping into the field like mobile phones locating their own specific satellites in space to download signals.

Certainly, after a year or so of working with the threshold field, many of the students had expanded their individual frequencies so much that they were able to break through the 'crystal ceiling' and see with their own eyes the vast new high-energy grids that we were accessing. This was wondrous work, but there was a price to pay. It left us all exhausted and fragile, sometimes for weeks on end. Clearly we needed to slow down and learn how to work with this new energy properly.

Grounding it proved to be essential; if we didn't, it literally flew around, causing exhaustion and chaos. This is why the *magi* and witches of the past had their staffs and broomsticks: they are a vital way of grounding the energy, fixing it back into the earth. Working at the sacred threshold demands the mastery and knowledge of energy demonstrated by these wise people of former times.

When we are working at this level, the sacred threshold may suddenly appear and open up spontaneously. This reminds me of the bit in *Harry Potter* where Harry is trying to find the platform for the train that will take him to his new school. He faces a blank wall where Platform 9¾ should be until the mother of another student gives him some advice, encouraging him to run right towards the platform (*the threshold*), promising that it will yield when he gets to it.

Like Platform 9¾, the sacred threshold is the opening between one landing and another. There could be several of these thresholds, as according to quantum physicists, there could be as many as ten dimensions of reality within our universe, all based on the varying energy levels that exist.

Interestingly, the threshold field is widening so much now that my current students are able to see it much sooner than their predecessors.

However you see the sacred threshold, you will be struck by its vastness, and a sense of altered time and unfamiliar boundaries that don't relate to any other physical or spiritual boundaries. It is magnificent – but not in any way compatible with life on this plane.

STANDING ON THE THRESHOLD

Towards the end, the dying enter this threshold space. All their senses become super-sensitive and they may become aware of worlds beyond this one. They often experience hallucinations, visits from deceased loved ones and prophetic dreams.

Catherine had been in the hospice for several weeks, hardly speaking, but when I went in to see her, she told me that her (deceased) parents and sister (a twin who had died at birth) were with her in the room. She carried on a detailed conversation with them while I was there.

Margaret, another dying friend, told me in great detail what was happening the following week – she said she had been there. She died soon afterwards, but everything she described actually did occur.

What does this show us about the true nature of time and the ability of consciousness to travel across different dimensions? Perhaps the threshold is a mystery that is designed to be beyond our reach...

AS DEATH APPROACHES

As death approaches, you will become aware of the energy shifting. If you have been working with your friend for a while, you will have observed the process of the elements withdrawing. Also, you may have noticed that your friend has been spending moments, or even long periods, outside their body. It is as if the dying practise what it is like to leave the constraints of the physical body behind. You will know they are approaching the sacred threshold.

Affirmation at the Sacred Threshold

Here is a prayer for peace, ease and grace at the sacred threshold:

> I offer my body up with gratitude for my life.
> I ask for my soul to travel with ease and grace during this transition.
> I ask for divine assistance at this most sacred time.
> May my heart be filled with love.
> May this love overflow and bring peace to my family and friends.
> I wish nothing but unconditional love to all.
> Ease, grace and love flow to me and through me.
> Amen
>
> **ELIZABETH HORNBY**

At this point the friend's lightbody will expand and their physical essence contract. Silence noisy machinery, switch off phones and dim the lights, if you have not done so already. Remove all sensory stimulants from the room just before transition to prevent any attachment to the Earth plane.

Act with simplicity, dignity and grace and set the tone by speaking quietly and behaving respectfully. Create an intention for love, calmness and an honouring of the friend who is passing. If in doubt about what to do, hold back for a while and ask yourself, *What would love do now?* Become very present and mindful: you are there as a witness and guardian to the subtle energy changes within your friend. It is your sacred role to lovingly assist by holding the space for whatever needs to unfold.

This can be a long session of waiting, watching and knowing. Practise deep listening (*see page 66*) and check that you are centred and grounded and feeling secure.

Family members may well look to you for guidance and support at this time. Sometimes they may want to be proactive in anointing and hand-holding, but at other times they may like you to take the lead and to witness the transition in their own space. Reassure them that they do not even need to be in the room if they choose not to be, but that you will be there so that their loved one won't be alone.

You may intuitively find yourself entering the dream state of your friend (*see pages 99–105*) and being able to guide them on their way. Whisper in their ear to follow the light, and let them know they will be greeted by someone who will come especially to meet them.

A death-rattle may occur as liquid gathers in the throat and chest. This sounds unpleasant but isn't usually distressing to the dying person. Reassure loved ones that this is just part of the process. Soothe and calm your dying friend by singing their name and assuring them that all is well.

Be mindful of your friend and everything they are experiencing, both physically and spiritually. They may begin to panic as they struggle to get enough oxygen; they may have a strong fear of an enveloping darkness, and they may feel resistant to letting go and surrendering.

You can help by:

- gently encouraging them to let go of their breath – use your mirrored breathing technique here (*see page 134*) and slowly ease the breath

- telling them how much they are loved and how much they have been loved

- reminding them that it is safe to go (give them permission if you feel that will help)

- reassuring them that they won't be alone; that there is no need to be frightened and that they will be loved and greeted as they make the transition.

Eventually you will sense a feeling of peace as they loosen their grasp on life.

Cultural and Religious Beliefs

It is worth noting a few important factors in relation to different faiths at the time of death, in case you are called by a hospice or care home to work with a friend at the last minute before their loved ones arrive. Always ask the hospice staff if they know if the dying friend has a particular faith.

Buddhism

Buddhists believe that when they die they will be born again. Their goal is to escape this cycle of death and rebirth and attain Nirvana, a state of perfect peace.

The state of mind of the dying person is very significant: a peaceful passing is thought to promote a joyful rebirth.

Buddhists believe that the spirit may take several days to leave the physical body, and that therefore the body should rest after death for three days and be treated with the greatest respect.

Christianity

Christians believe that they will go to heaven once they have died. You could recite the Lord's Prayer as the person passes.

Catholics believe that they will see God face to face at the moment of death. They also believe that they must repent of their sins in order to enter the full glory of heaven. When a person is close to death, the family or friends will ask a priest to come and pray with the sick person, and the Sacrament of the Anointing of the Sick is administered. This includes anointing with Holy Oils and receiving the Sacrament of Penance and Reconciliation and Holy Communion.

Hinduism

Because Hindus believe in reincarnation, they see death as a soul merely moving forwards on the path towards heaven (Nirvana).

Avoid touching the body once death has occurred. The family will pray around the body soon after death.

Islam

Muslim customs may vary depending on the type of faith: Shi'ite or Sunni Muslims accept death as Allah's will and prepare for it with daily prayers. A dying person may wish to face Mecca.

Many Muslims believe that by accepting Islam, even just before death, and saying the Shahaadah (a declaration of faith), the dying person will go to Jannah (heaven) after death.

After death, the eyes should be closed and the body turned to face Mecca. Family members will wash the body and wrap it in a shroud. Burial should take place within 24 hours.

Judaism

Jews believe that when they die they will go to heaven to be with God. This next world is called Olam HaEmet, the World of Truth. Death is seen as a part of life and a part of God's plan.

Beliefs may vary according to whether the person is Orthodox, Reform or Conservative. In any event, a rabbi should be called.

At the time of death, the person's eyes are closed, the body is covered and laid on the floor and candles are lit. The body should never be left unattended until a rabbi or loved ones arrive. Eating and drinking are not allowed near the body as a sign of respect. Washing of the body is considered a sacred act and should only be performed by specific members of the Jewish community. Burial should take place as soon as possible after death.

Sikhism

Sikhs view death as a separation of the soul from the body. It is considered to be God's will. Sikhs believe that the soul moves on to meet the supreme soul, God. Death is seen as a time for praising God in accordance with the teachings of the code of conduct, the Rahit Maryada.

When someone dies, if the body is on a bed it should not be moved and no light should be placed next to it. Prayers are said which acknowledge that the death is an act of God.

Seeing the Spirit Leave

Soul Midwives sometimes see the soul or spirit energy leave the body before clinical death has been recorded. Perhaps this is because the work here is done and the soul and spirit have crossed the threshold before the body has caught up. You can feel them shift and leave, with all the energetic effects of crossing the threshold (*see below*), even though the person's heart is still beating and they are continuing to breathe.

AT THE TIME OF DEATH

There are powerful forces at work at this time. Be aware that just before the last intake of breath, but not necessarily at the point of death, the soul goes into a place of unconditional love and has the opportunity to deal with any unfinished business while often experiencing a series of life reviews. This is a very reverent and sacred time, and it is important that the Soul Midwife ensures, as far as possible, that the dying space is peaceful and sacrosanct.

The dying friend will begin a rapid expansion into awareness, and as they take their last breath you will sense their body emptying and becoming a hollow vessel as the remaining life force ebbs away. (Note that if your friend's breathing has become very irregular you may not be immediately aware of the last breath.)

As death occurs, the spirit detaches from the body with a rapid sense of upward flight, like a balloon taking off. The shift of energy can be very dramatic – an energy explosion creating shockwaves around the room.

The sacred threshold feels exquisitely light and claustrophobically dense; it is illuminated yet heavy – and both ecstatic and sombre. It is a very seductive place, with extraordinary energies to which you can easily become attached. Do not attempt to journey with your friend to this place unless you are well grounded and trained in this deep esoteric work. If you wish to help your friend as they cross the threshold, being very present and honouring their journey is enough.

Soul Midwives may experience the light energy moving through them at this time. This can be alarming and can make you feel restless and anxious. It may hit your blockages (commonly in the solar plexus) and you may feel a tightening and discomfort in three centres: the throat, the solar plexus and the anal region. You may also feel an expanding and awakening in your heart space, and warmth there, as if warm water is starting to flow in and out of your heart area. Your soul may be resonating with the departing soul, perhaps as part of your own learning process.

This entire process of transformation expands our energy dramatically for a short burst, but as it decreases again, it can make us feel exhausted and even cause temporary pains in the body. The energy explosion as the person departs is often followed by a vacuum-like force which sucks the energy from the room, including the warmth. A sudden chill can appear and the area around the dead friend can feel very cold. A brooding, restless cloud of chaotic darkness descends. This is the doldrums of the deep soul – the bottom of its ocean bed as it tethers itself to eternity.

More medical indicators of death are:

- outward gasps as the heart and lungs cease to function

- a long out-breath, followed a few seconds later by what appears to be another intake of breath but is actually the lungs expelling air

- no pulse

- the skin colour swiftly changing to sallow yellow

- the facial expression altering or slackening.

At the immediate time of death, take the time to be quiet around the person who has died. Connect with them and explain that you understand that they are merging with the light and are now released from their body. Offer to be there to give love and understanding for as long as is needed. Mark their passing with a simple ceremony, such as a prayer or the lighting of a candle, and tell them that you will keep a candle lit to light their way as they journey. They are not alone, but held in love.

Helen Fields e-mailed me from Cyprus, describing her profound experience when her son died:

> When Chris... was in the intensive care unit (he had a brain injury) I realized I had a choice of how to deal with the situation: either open my heart or close it. So it was not really a choice – I had to open my heart for myself and my family and for all the young people around me.
>
> Since his death – which was very peaceful, and my father was waiting for Chris to help him pass – I have called the whole episode 'Divine Order'. It was as though it was all laid out; we just had to be open and follow the lead.
>
> The intensive care staff at Bath hospital were wonderful. There must have been about 40 young people around Chris's bed the evening before his life support was turned off, and they beat drum rhythms on their chests and wrists to say their farewells. Chris was a samba drummer in his spare time.
>
> My sister and I opened the sacred space and all the time talked to him and gave him the choice to stay or go. It was such a shock for us all, but so beautiful as well. He was ready to go and his heart stopped after 10 minutes. He was ready to donate (he donated his heart valves, liver, kidneys, cornea, and for research, his pancreas) and the surgery went very well.

Death can be a special moment. Nurses, doctors, chaplains and those who care for the dying brim with stories of mysterious coincidences, deathbed experiences, premonitions, visions, auras and the amazing energy felt in the room as a person dies.

These phenomena are different from the 'near-death' sensations of bright lights and tunnels reported by those who recover from trauma or cardiac arrest. These quiet, everyday experiences of the dying have an intrinsically transcendental quality which is deeply human.

Nina was asked to sit with an old lady who was alone:

I must admit, as I sat in her room, on her bed, with the scent of the freesia perfume she wore still lingering, I cried. There was something so sad about being the only person there, and I was a complete stranger.

Where were all her relatives and friends? Dead, I supposed.

Then something strange happened. A blackbird tapped on the window several times. It flew back and forth but kept coming back and tapping. I just knew that this bird had come to fetch her. Perhaps it was her mother or father, or an angel – I don't know, but it felt very special.

AFTER DEATH

Closing the Sacred Space

Working at the sacred threshold is an honour and requires an acknowledgement of sacred duty. Be led by your heart and intuition as to when to close the space and be silent.

You may wish to close the sacred space with the following words:

South, West, North and East,
Thank you for holding this space in peace.
Earth below and sky above,
Thank you for holding this space in Love.

CHARLOTTE GUSH

You might also like to give the friend assurances directly as they go through the process of separating spirit and soul from their body. Acknowledge that they are on their way; that they no longer need their body and are embarking on a greater journey.

Gently talk loved ones through what happens next. Many people feel that they must call the undertaker straight away, but reassure them that they can take their time if they want to. They should not feel rushed into saying goodbye too quickly, as it is something that may cause regret later on. Encourage gentle conversation around the body.

The Separation of Spirit and Soul

Soon after clinical death, the final stage (the separation of spirit and soul) will take place.

This is an energetic event which can be intuited and sometimes seen. It is the separation of a thin silver cord which spins from a centre point in two opposite directions. The spinning motion thins the cord, which dissolves and separates the body and spirit soul. Once this has happened, transition has fully taken place.

Some Soul Midwives in ancient times actually participated in this separation by cutting or blowing the cord. Small sickle-shaped implements, feathers, or simply the breath was used.

Bringing Yourself Back into Balance

After sacred work, especially facilitating transition, you will have generated a great deal of energy. Try not to hug or touch people until you have sealed your aura and restored your balance. (This can be very difficult if you are comforting relatives, who will themselves be very affected by such a profound experience.)

You can bring yourself back into balance by:

- grounding and centring yourself (the easiest way is by sitting quietly and focusing on your own breathing whilst consciously grounding your energy back into the earth)

- cleansing your energy fields so they are sparkling clean (starting at your crown chakra, move your intention down your body, clearing and sealing your field as you go)

- closing your chakras down to a practical level to stop your energy leaking. Do this by starting at your feet and imagining each chakra through your body as semi-open. It may help to see the chakras as lotus flowers which have just started to open.

- re-energizing your fields to help them come back into balance. Here again, check your chakras to see that they are all half open, and also check that your aura feels strong and healthy by picturing an invisible membrane around you which is strong and intact. If you sense any holes where energy may be leaking, imagine stretching the membrane across the hole and sealing it back together again.

- replenishing your reserves of energy so that you aren't running on empty

- protecting yourself from any unwelcome etheric parasites or spirit attachments. Do this by asking your guides to free you of attachments, or use Soul Midwife prayer beads as an exercise to clear yourself after working (*see pages 218 and 254*).

You may feel the spirit of your friend around you for some time after the death. It can be hours or days, but usually it takes about three days for the energy signature to disperse. If you experience a sense of your friend, continue to talk to them and reassure them as they move towards the light. Light a candle for them and say prayers.

Many traditions recognize the period of resting between death and burial as sacred, and there are many rituals which honour this time.

Practical Considerations after Death

After death, there are several ways in which a Soul Midwife can help:

- washing/preparing the body

- advising on formalities relating to documentation

- helping with funeral arrangements

Washing / Preparing the Body

If a patient dies in hospital, washing and preparing the body will be taken care of by the nursing staff. If the friend has died at home, you may be asked by the family to help with the final preparations. Washing and preparing a body for burial can be one of the most devotional acts of love you can perform.

HOW TO PREPARE THE BODY

- ✎ Close the eyes.

- ✎ If the friend wore dentures, insert them (it is easier to do this before rigor mortis has taken effect).

- ✎ If you wish, wrap gauze around the head – from the top of the head and under the chin – in order to keep the mouth shut prior to rigor mortis.

- ❧ Cleanse the body (you will not usually be required to prepare the body fully before the undertaker arrives, but it can help relatives if the hands and face have been washed and any secretions from the eyes, nose and mouth cleared).

- ❧ Comb the hair and make it tidy.

- ❧ Adjust the bed so that it is entirely flat. Straighten the linen and then pull the deceased's arms out so they are lying outside the blanket or duvet, straight at each side of the body. Hands should be accessible for family members to reach out and touch.

Blessings

During the washing and preparation of the body, blessings can be said to honour your friend.

Here is a Soul Midwife's blessing:

May peace surround you.

May light shine within you.

May your soul be held in love.

Anointing

You may have already agreed with your friend and their loved ones that you will anoint the body. The symbolic meaning of anointing at this time is to prepare and nourish the soul for its onward journey.

Anoint your friend on the same points as before death (*see pages 126–128*). Soul Midwives usually use fragonia or rose oil to anoint a body. Rigor mortis begins to set in between two and four hours after death, so anointing should be done before then.

Also conduct any ritual or religious customs in accordance with the friend's wishes. Create a sanctuary space with soft lighting, preferably candlelight, and quiet music.

Documentation

The procedures for this will be different across the world, and you will need to check on the current requirements in order to work within regional legalities.

Wherever you are, if your friend dies at home, record the time of death and notify a doctor. In the UK, there is no requirement to call the undertaker immediately. Unless there is to be a postmortem examination, the body can remain at home or in a place of rest until the funeral. As a general rule, the friend may be left to rest for up to three days after death before being moved or disturbed. This rule can vary according to different religious and cultural customs (*see pages 174–176*).

Following a death in the UK, there are certain formalities which must be completed in the first few days:

- get a death certificate – this will be from a doctor (GP or at a hospital). It is required in order to register the death.

- register the death within five days – this provides the relevant documents required for a funeral

- arrange the funeral – loved ones can use a funeral director or arrange the funeral themselves

BRINGING CLOSURE

After working with a friend and their family, you will eventually need to bring closure to the relationship. It may help to ask yourself the following questions:

- 'Did I actively help my friend to achieve the death they hoped for?'

- 'Did I help my friend to express their individual wishes, rather than my own idea of what those wishes might have been?'

- 'Did I look at all the other resources that were available to them, such as including their family, friends, organizations, etc?'

- 'Did I act at all times with deep respect for my friend, facilitate equal partnership in our work together and show willingness to go the extra mile?'

Most Soul Midwives meet the families of their friends a month or so after the death to find out how they are, share experiences and talk over the death if necessary, refer them for bereavement help if required, and sometimes to hold a simple blessing ceremony to bring closure.

Visits from Beyond the Threshold

It's not only Soul Midwives who meet the families afterwards. Many families who are newly grieving receive signs – sometimes subtle, sometimes not – that their loved ones are present.

These often manifest in the form of birds, butterflies or animals acting strangely. I have lost count of how many stories I have heard about birds flying into the house and staying around for a few days following a death, or a cat arriving, or a pet behaving differently. I once heard of an out-of-season butterfly that seemed to be everywhere, fluttering around the supper table and even appearing at the funeral.

Sometimes, a particular perfume will linger in the house. Once, after a death, a colleague woke up to find single flowers placed around the house.

The strangest story I heard was the appearance on a bedroom wall of a message written in lipstick after the sudden death of a young husband. It simply said, 'I love you.'

SUMMARY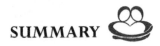

- The sacred threshold is the boundary between life and death.

- Working at the sacred threshold is an honour and requires an acknowledgement of your sacred duty. Be led by your heart and intuition.

- Create a sacred cocoon for the friend as they approach the threshold.

- Be present and mindful and reassure them that they are loved and safe.

- Hold the sacred space for them as they cross the threshold.

- Mark their passing with a simple ritual such as a prayer or the lighting of a candle.

- Afterwards, reassure the family.

- Close the sacred space.

- Look after yourself and take some time to revitalize your own energy.

- Wash, prepare and anoint the body if requested.

- Complete the practical formalities in relation to a death, e.g. recording the time of death.

- Later, visit the family to bring closure.

- Be open to contact from the departed friend.

❧ PART III ❧
THE SOUL MIDWIFE'S
TOOL KIT

'The eye of the vision is within the soul.

Let those who have the vision see.

Those that would listen let them hear.'

Gospel of Mary Magdalene

CHAPTER 10

TOOLS

'Whether the plant is to heal the body or the spirit...
what makes it work is your good intention towards the plant.
They are beings which have their own forms, or they can be like
human beings with faces and bodies.When the spirit accepts the person,
and the person has the will, the spirit grants them energy.
The path to knowledge opens, and the healing takes place.'
GUILLERMO ARÉVALO, A SHIPIBO MAESTRO

I live within a bowl of hills, a hollow within a grand formation of ancient rocks on southern England's Jurassic coast. The landscape is strewn with covered green lanes which used to connect the tiny hamlets and villages before the roads were built. Some of these lanes are literally thousands of years old and are full of wild plants and trees that have never been touched by fertilizers or chemicals of any kind. These hedgerows contain almost everything for a Soul Midwife's pharmacopeia. From my front door I can stretch out an arm and pick bunches of marzipan-scented meadowsweet (beloved by the Druids for its ability to cure everything from diarrhoea to depression), tender green nettles, yellow archangel, lemon balm and water mint, while the orchard beside the house has a collection of gnarled old fruit trees and also hawthorn, mistletoe, hazel, witch hazel, alder and willow. In the old herb patch there is always angelica, lemon verbena, rosemary, thyme, roses, nasturtiums, chamomile and marigolds. And tucked safely away in a dark and hidden place behind a stone wall where the grass snakes live, there are the wise-crone plants: monkshood, foxglove, aconite, yew, henbane, comfrey, woad, artemisia and lady's mantle.

I have worked with herbs, plants, mosses and oils all my life. In my straw-bale apothecary, which is down amongst the apple trees, I make remedies in the traditional way. I have an almanac that predicts the best time to do this, as some days of the year are more potent than others for making essences. For example, the new moon, full moon, solstices, eclipses and equinoxes are when the energies are at their strongest.

The wise men and women who used to live around here, the cunning folk as they were called, were the Soul Midwives of their time and concocted herbal remedies to heal village folk from cradle to grave. They could turn their hands to making cures for almost anything. They were skilled at working simple folk magic too. They used divination – often scrying (seeing) in water – to see if there was a curse behind a mystery illness, or why a local cow was producing sour milk. In Cornwall, where I was born, they were sometimes called *pellars*, a name thought to be derived from 'the expellers' because they were often called to expel evil spirits.

Modern drugs have, of course, done away with the need for most of these old remedies. But sometimes, in the early stages of illness, just as the symptoms are becoming troublesome, drugs can be a little too strong and can cause unwelcome side-effects. For this reason it is useful to have some knowledge of herbal lore and other preparations that can help a dying friend.

Also, apart from the gentle teas and tinctures described in this chapter, Soul Midwives never give remedies to be taken internally. Instead they will use them as aura rubs or sprinkle them into the friend's navel (a natural container for vibrational essences).

HERBS

Herb teas can occasionally be helpful to the dying. German chamomile and lemon balm, for example, are two herbs that reduce nausea and inflammation, as they help to relax the stomach. In the old days, dandelion root was the cottage cure for diarrhoea and vomiting. The fresh leaves were crushed and added to soups. Cinnamon in milk can also help the digestion.

Many of my friends have found ginger tea wonderful for easing nausea. All you need to do is infuse one fresh chopped ginger root in a cup of hot water for 15 minutes. You can take this with food or by the spoonful.

Aloe vera juice is very helpful for the painful mouth ulcers that appear during chemotherapy.

A coffee tincture made from mixing ¼ teaspoon of coffee granules with 1 tablespoon of clear spirits (i.e. vodka or brandy) can be used as an aura wash (on the hands of the Soul Midwife) or placed in the friend's tummy button cavity to help when they are moving from one stage to another.

FLOWER REMEDIES

Flower remedies work very well for some people and are easy to make. If I am making them for a friend, I will look at what plants are growing in or around their garden and see if they'll be useful.

On summer mornings I pick the blooms and leaves shortly after sunrise before soaking them in spring water (or water from the little silver river Winnaford that flows at the bottom of our land).

The flowers are then left out in the sunshine to absorb the warmth and light before being decanted into mother stock bottles and fixed with a little apple brandy.

Each plant has a resonance with a particular element, time of year or disease, so there are many correspondences to work with.

The mother tinctures seem to hold their energy for two or three years, but if I run out, I also use the Bach Flower Remedies. I would never be without:

- Crab Apple – for when friends are feeling toxic, especially after chemotherapy

- Elm – for when friends are feeling completely overwhelmed by their situation

- Olive – for exhaustion

- Sweet Chestnut – for anxious thoughts

VIBRATIONAL REMEDIES

I also make more unusual vibrational remedies when particular weather conditions prevail, such as thunder and lightning, storms, snow, extreme heat, humidity, excessive rain and howling autumn gales.

These remedies contain bottled life force which is both primal and elemental. All of them carry the vibration of the element involved, and they can be very useful for treating friends as the elements withdraw during the active stage.

For instance, a vibrational remedy made from snowflakes that have melted and turned into water would be an excellent treatment for all stages of transition, as its key energy would be in matter changing form.

Vibrational remedies are also wonderful for moving both Soul Midwife and friend out of melancholy or a gloomy mood. A few drops of autumn wind can shift you out of lethargy, as well as help a friend ease through the Air stage (*see Resources*).

ESSENTIAL OILS

The following recipes, which all include essential oils, are ideal for the Soul Midwife tool kit:

Therapeutic Touch Hand Massage Cream

To make the hand cream:

- Add a 60 ml (2 oz) jar of beeswax to a ⅓ mixture of shea butter and/or coconut oil with ⅓ extra virgin olive oil.

- Microwave the mixture in five-second bursts until it has melted.

- When it is cool, add a few drops of lavender oil.

Mildly Medicated Handwash

This handwash is ideal to use after any bodywork. The following quantities make approximately 1 litre (1½ pints) of solution:

- Mix together one part aloe vera gel to six parts cooled boiled water.

- Add three tablespoons of calendula oil and a few drops of tea tree oil and lavender oil. Shake well.

- Store in a glass bottle with a pump top.

Massage Oil

This massage oil is ideal for very dry, cracked skin (particularly after the Fire stage). It is made from a mixture of the following ingredients:

- 2 drops of eucalyptus essential oil

- 3 drops of clary sage essential oil

- 5 drops of geranium/Egyptian essential oil

- 5 drops of bergamot essential oil

- 15 drops of lavender essential oil

- 20mls (0.7 fl.oz) of carrot tissue oil

- Mix the oils together and store in a glass bottle.

Lip Balm

This can be very soothing when lips are very dry and cracking.

- Melt together 1 teaspoon cocoa butter, 1 teaspoon beeswax and 30mls (1 fl.oz) of sweet almond oil.

- Add 6 drops of your preferred essential oil.

- Store in a glass pot and keep cool.

PLANT OILS

Many years ago I was given knowledge of the myrrhophore tradition – a way of working with plant oils dating back to Egyptian times. There are very few practitioners working in this traditional way today, but it has so many applications, especially with the dying.

Much of the myrrhophore tradition is linked with the Jewish esoteric teachings of the Kabbalah, and the oils are sacred tools used in deep soul work such as:

- reconnecting with the lightbody

- connecting with the Shekinah – the intuitive, sacred feminine aspect of the divine that exists within all of us

- absorbing the divine breath for the onward journey of the soul

- merging the soul with the universe

- healing karmic soul wounds

- working with the life between lives

Some of the oils have peculiar names, smell strange and are extremely costly and hard to source. However, acquiring them is worth the effort and expense, as they work on a very deep level of spirit and soul. Their energy fields vibrate at a frequency high enough to resonate with the lightbody, making them powerful tools for the physical body and, more importantly, the super-consciousness.

I think these oils contain a 'God' particle and are carriers of pure life force. They work in conjunction with specific energy points in the body. Some of them are so potent that they need to be kept in the dark and well away from electromagnetic fields.

Some of the oils in this category are angelica, kewra, ravensara and violet (which is almost impossible to obtain). However, one of the most beautiful oils I work with is very easily made and comes from the fragrant red juice of the flowers of St John's wort. It is said to resemble the blood and wounds of Jesus Christ. It is the best wound oil I know of, and as well as soothing pain, it is anti-inflammatory and healing.

Jesus Oil (St John's Wort Oil)

For wound healing and pressure sores.

- Pick the flowers of St John's wort on a sunny day.

- Place the flowers loosely in a bottle and completely cover them with a fine organic olive oil.

- Leave the bottle to stand in the sun for a few weeks.

- After a time the oil will become red. Strain through muslin and store in dark bottles.

- To prepare an infusion, add 1 heaped teaspoon per ¼ litre (½ pint) of boiling water and infuse for a short time.

Hydrolats

Unlike essential oils, hydrolats are fairly unstable and must be kept refrigerated to prevent spoilage. If properly stored, most have a shelf life of one to two years. They are cheaper to purchase than essential oils. (*See pages 123–124 for a list of hydrolats recommended for use with the dying.*)

TOOLS FOR VIGILING

Singing Bowls

If I know that I shall be vigiling for someone, I pack my singing bowls in my bag. Their gentle tones are soft, sonorous and beautiful, and as well as helping people to relax, they can restore balance and intensify consciousness. Their vibrations help the soul to move in and out of the body, and they are increasingly being played in hospices to soften the death process. In the East, they are used to create a sacred space before prayer or meditation and to prepare people before they begin specific spiritual exercises.

I work with separate singing bowls, as each bowl has a different personality. My big bowl, which I struggle to hold in my hand because it's so large and heavy, is tuned to the heart chakra. It is a good general bowl to use in any situation.

My next bowl, which is smaller, has been created with the specific intention of working with the broken-hearted – those filled with grief or deep inner soul wounds which they are finding hard to heal.

And my smallest bowl, which I found on a junk stall at a market, has a sweetness about it and an affinity with putting people's minds and hearts at rest. It somehow helps them to lay down their weariness and let go of their worries. It works particularly well with people who are in the pre-active stage and have just been told that they are terminally ill.

Sometimes I ring my bowls with a muted suede mallet, and at other times I strike them with a felt-topped baton, which produces a softer and longer tone. It doesn't really matter how they are played, as their vibrations are somehow felt in the bones and they fill the room with love and peace. I find that a session of about 30 minutes is usually quite long enough to promote healing and tranquillity.

Certain notes have an affinity with certain chakras, and sound waves spread into the room like concentric rings from a stone dropped into a pond, widening out into larger and larger circles. These sound ripples pass through blood, flesh, organs and even bones, relaxing them and at the same time harmonizing and energizing them.

In a sound bath session, where you can work with a number of different instruments (tingshas, chimes, rain sticks etc.), you will be giving 100 billion cells in the human body a gentle massage. This will usually soothe away pain and fear and leave the friend feeling very relaxed.

One night I was asked if I would bring my bowls to play for Josh, who was in a hospice. I had met him several times over the previous few years as he had been a pioneering sound practitioner before he had fallen ill. He knew exactly what to expect from a sound bath and asked for certain bowls to be placed on top of his chest and stomach so that he could feel the vibrations and absorb the sound.

The session started with some hands-on healing. When Josh felt settled, I started to play the bowls, ringing them so that their vibrations and sounds merged together. I carried on for about 20 minutes, and finished, when I saw he was tiring, by striking the two smallest bowls at the same time and then bringing them together, bowl to bowl, over his heart.

The sound waves danced around him and Josh closed his eyes and slipped into a very peaceful meditative state. As he dropped deeper and deeper into himself, his aura changed colour and became a beautiful mirage of greens, heavenly blues and turquoise, edged with gold.

He fell asleep and I left quietly, noticing that his breathing was shallow but very peaceful.

A nurse called later to say that he had died peacefully in his sleep four hours later. It seems that his struggle to let go may have been eased by the singing bowls, and his body and soul were able to loosen their binds to each other.

Please note that singing bowls should not be used too close to death, or if the friend is confused, hallucinating or agitated.

Music

Not all of us feel confident making music and playing instruments ourselves. If it's just not your thing, having a comprehensive selection of suitable CDs is a very good substitute (*see pages 154–155*).

Comfort Items

Comfort items may include:

- The Soul Midwives' symbol to hang on the door (*you can see this on the front cover of this book above the two figures*).This shows that a Soul Midwife is vigiling and that privacy and quiet are required.

- A comfort blanket or shawl to swaddle the dying person. Most Soul Midwives have a range of pastel-coloured woollen or mohair blankets and ask friends to choose which they'd prefer (interestingly, most people choose a pale pink one).

- Soft toys and teddy bears. These can be very comforting for the dying person to hold or be tucked up with. Charity shops are a great source of cuddly animals. When you leave a friend with a cuddly toy, it's theirs forever. Some people find their cuddly animal so comforting that they ask to be buried with it.

- Talisman stones. Many friends find that a smooth polished stone such as rose quartz or amethyst can be soothing and comforting to hold. Often the Soul Midwife will imbue the stone with healing energy by transferring energy into it which can then be absorbed when it is held.

CLEANING OUR TOOLS

Everything we use (including ourselves) when working with a friend may absorb the vibration of the friend and also their illness, which is why we need to apply strict spiritual hygiene measures. It is extremely important to clean your tools after a session with a friend, whether those tools are a singing bowl, tuning fork, essential oils or even your hands.

Here are some simple ways of cleaning tools:

- putting items in sunlight for a few hours

- burning sage. (Sage has a natural aroma to it that repels negative energy. It is said that ghosts and lower entities cannot be around this smell. Smudging – wafting burning sage – in a room and over your body and tools is a wonderful way to end a session with a friend if lots of energy has been moved.)

- leaving your tools out, or going out yourself, in the light of the full moon

- being spritzed with healing water or holy water

- washing yourself or your tools in the ocean, or sitting near it for some time

- soaking your tools in saltwater or laying them out on a plate of salt

- simply being in nature

All these methods are healing and cleansing. Find out which work for you and keep yourself and your tools clean. Remember, when you are a healer, you do have to cleanse and protect yourself (*see also Chapter 11*), and these methods will also keep your energy pure to assist your friends.

SUMMARY

Here are some suggestions for the contents of your Soul Midwife's tool kit or medicine bag:

- wax battery-operated candles (available widely online) to bring a soft glow to the room or for ritual and blessings; these are completely safe to use, and pose no fire risk

- CDs of soothing music

- a CD player or iPod dock

- essential oils – an assortment is good, but always include fragonia, frankincense, rose and sandalwood

- hydrolats – these are gentler than pure essential oils

- soft blankets for swaddling – use colours such as pale pink, aqua, gold and pale green

- cuddly toys

- musical instruments – singing bowls, harps, lyres, simple percussive instruments and wind chimes for giving simple sound baths

- an energy chime bar for diagnostic use

- homoeopathic remedies

- flower remedies – either homemade or bought

- base oils such as grapeseed or avocado for massaging hands and feet

- a memory-foam cushion for use when massaging hands and feet

- chocolate, etc. (emergency rations for Soul Midwives!); also a Thermos flask, herbal teabags and biscuits

- a torch or book light

- air fresheners

- coffee tincture (*see page 193*)

- homoeopathic strength ayahuasca water (for psychopomp work)

- Bach Flower Remedies – useful remedies are Water Violet, Impatiens (for agitation and restlessness) and Elm and Sweet Chestnut (for uncontrolled and disturbing thoughts).

CHAPTER 11

SELF-CARE

'Compassion is not a relationship between the healer and the
wounded. It's a relationship between equals. Only when we know our
own darkness well can we be present with the darkness of others.
Compassion becomes real when we recognize our shared humanity.'

PEMA CHÖDRÖN

People who are attracted to Soul Midwifery desire to be of service, and to become a conduit of healing light. The work certainly gives us glimpses of paradise, but there are also pitfalls. There is no light without the dark. This is, after all, the cosmic law of balance.

The connections we make with our friends are deep and profound, but they are not necessarily divine. The dying don't suddenly change into angels just because they are on their way to heaven. Also, being surrounded by the energy of someone who is dying can be very exhausting. It has a peculiar feel to it – a bit like a caffeine rush. Emotions can range from extreme anxiety to anger and weepiness, and Soul Midwives can end up completely drained.

We must be careful not to absorb the pain or suffering of our friends to a point where it affects us. This is intense work and we have to keep a healthy balance and ensure we are truly living our own lives.

CLEANSING AND PROTECTION

We need to be protected and practise good spiritual hygiene when we are involved in any kind of healing work, and Soul Midwifery is no exception.

As we may absorb the energy and illness of our friends and their families unknowingly as we work with them, we need to be very vigilant about cleansing both ourselves and our tools.

CLEANSING AND PROTECTION WHEN WORKING WITH FRIENDS

- ❧ Place a large bowl of water with a handful of salt in the room where you will be working. This will aid in absorbing the negative energy from any of the session.

- ❧ Wear neutral or darker colours at the bedside. Many of us like to wear soft pastel colours, but pale colours tend to absorb energy. If you are feeling at all stressed, tired or out of balance, wear something darker to protect yourself from any low-vibrational energy.

- ❧ Wearing purple or a purple amethyst pendant can serve to block any oncoming negative energy. Purple is the colour of protection and spiritual healing. This is why Christian monks and Catholic priests would wear purple robes with hoods when in confession (release) chambers. These robes protected their entire body from negative energies and mental programmes.

- ❧ After sacred work, wash your hands. This immediately neutralizes attachment, especially if you have been working energetically with a friend. Fill a sink with cold water and add some essential oils – possibly lavender or rose to clear the energy (*see also below*). Liquid soap which has salt added is very useful.

- Singing and toning are good methods of releasing energy and rebalancing yourself after a healing session. Try singing alternating high and low notes as loudly as you can for a few minutes. This will clear any negative energy and help to rebalance the chakras, and the strength of your voice will also give you an indication of the strength of your own energy field. There are some very good toning CDs available which you can play and sing along with.

- Exercise is the very best way of neutralizing unharmonious energy. Walking, swimming and cycling are great ways of staying spiritually well.

- Cultivate a rebalancing meditation, such as Vipassana, where you untangle energy piece by piece throughout the body in order to burn off any residual threshold energy or cords (*see page 210*) that have formed during your work with your friend.

- If you are feeling toxic or overloaded, run a bath and fill it with natural sea salt or Epsom salts.

- Best of all, if it's warm, go for a swim in the sea!

Cleansing the Aura of the Feet and Legs with Essential Oils

There is a reason why the disciples would have cleansed Jesus' feet with water, and why people in India bless and the feet of their gurus: the feet and lower legs (below the knees) are where the body releases most of its energy. It is also where it can attract lots of energy from everywhere we walk. Cleansing this portion of the body serves to revitalize these energy pathways so that we're energetically moving again.

- Place a few drops of eucalyptus, palo santo, pemou (also known as Siam wood), sage or tea tree oil into a cup of water. You can even put a little salt into it.

- First wash your feet and lower legs with soap and water if you wish.

- Mix up the essential oil/water and pour some onto your hands.

- Rub your hands with this powerful tonic and then wash your feet and lower legs with it.

Revitalizing your Energy Field

Many Soul Midwives and healers (including me) have to spend long periods alone, away from company and often in complete silence in order to rebalance themselves after spiritual work.

The following oils are recommended for use by the Soul Midwife after working with a friend:

- Clove – clears the aura; a very powerful oil used in the myrrhophore tradition

- Fragonia – useful for Soul Midwives who are overcharged and exhausted

- Pemou – useful for cutting cords (*see page 210*) and karmic connections

EMPATHY AND SYMPATHY

Some Soul Midwives tune in so deeply to the inner processes of others that they often experience telepathy or insights into the future or past lives of their friends. At times it can be hard to distinguish between our 'stuff' and the friend's issues. Our identities can merge and boundaries become blurred.

Accomplished shamans, psychics and spiritual healers can enter these deep states safely, but usually only after years of practice. Inexperienced people undertaking deep work of any kind, let alone in the maelstrom of energies surrounding the dying, may sometimes experience disturbing psychic crises. So it is important to develop the work slowly and safely and not be tempted to go out of our depth.

We have to be total masters of ourselves when we work with these energies, and ensure that we close down again by consciously closing our chakras (*see pages 106–111*) from head to toe after a healing session.

COMPASSION FATIGUE

We need to have compassion for ourselves in order to be able to help others. If you are feeling sad and exhausted and are suffering from compassion fatigue:

- Take time out to rest. See friends, but seek healing time alone as well. Allow yourself to slow down and don't try to do too much too quickly.

- Take care of yourself by eating, resting, sleeping and exercising. Cry when you need to and share your feelings with those you are close to or a Soul Midwife buddy or mentor.

- Give yourself a hand and foot massage with fragonia oil diluted in grapeseed oil.

- Try unwinding in a warm bath with Epsom salts.

- Listen to gentle music.

- Do some yoga or gentle stretching.

Dissolving the Cords

When we work with a friend, cords of energy flow between us. If we don't cut these cords after a session, every time the friend thinks about us, they may subconsciously be drawing energy from us, and we can quickly become drained.

- Make yourself comfortable and ensure that you won't be interrupted.

- Breathe very deeply, imagining that you are breathing out anything that no longer serves you.

- Starting from your head and going down to your toes, search for any cords of energy which are still linking you to your friend.

- Then ask that they be dissolved with love.

A useful affirmation after cutting the cords is something like:

'I release my friend and I dissolve all cords of attachment from us. We are both free from physical and karmic connection and continue with our lives separately.'

Relationships with certain friends can be further complicated by soul contracts between us, as well as karmic issues. If this is the case, take special care to cut the cords and release and neutralize the energy generated during a session.

EXERCISE **Lighting a Candle**

Another idea is to light a candle and use your intention to bless the friend, forgive yourself and forgive them for anything that has been previously spoken of, done or thought about in the past.

You may want to use the Ho'oponopono mantra from the shamanic practices native to Hawaii:

'I am sorry
Please forgive me
I love you
Thank you.'

Then close your chakras down (*see pages 106–111*), before imagining your friend filling with healing white light.

STAY GROUNDED

The whole territory of working with the dying is a rich energy matrix; add emotions, fear, shadow, anguish, soul wounds and projection and you can see why you need to keep your hat on and stay grounded.

Curanderismo, the folk medicine of South America, has a word, *susto*, to describe a type of panic attack which affects healers when they are overstressed and vulnerable due to exhaustion. *Susto* causes the soul to be knocked sideways out of the body. I have seen this in many Soul Midwives when they have been working too hard. The cure is to call the soul back in and then to perform a small healing ritual called a *limpias* (blessing) to cleanse and restore the mind, body and spirit. This is a very specific ritual which needs to be done by an experienced *curandero* using eggs as a medium for drawing out negativity. An experienced Soul Midwife would probably also be able to help a colleague.

Another condition that is common to soul workers is *accedie*, a state of spiritual dryness where life can seem dull and banal. This often happens after working in ecstatic states and can take away our appetite for life. As St John of the Cross said, 'Nothing worldly satisfies one who has tasted the Divine.' And yet, as one Zen master said, even after enlightenment, you still need to go out, chop wood and carry water.

Spiritual Emergencies

The more sensitive we become, the greater the discipline and awareness we need to develop. This requires going deeper within ourselves to become strong vessels to contain spirit. When we are tired or too open, or just inexperienced and ungrounded in our spiritual work, we can sometimes experience a spiritual emergency.

A spiritual emergency may be defined as a sudden shift, or opening out into a much higher vibration without any warning. While people are experiencing this, they are extremely sensitive to all psychic phenomena and may hear voices, see bright colours and be super-intuitive. They may feel completely overwhelmed and frightened by their experiences – or intrigued by them. As psychiatrist Stanislav Grof, an expert in the field of spiritual emergency, warns:

> *It is easy to become fascinated by the opening realm of psychic phenomena and interpret their occurrence as an indication of one's own superiority and special calling. Since the goal of the spiritual path is transcending the ego, such an attitude represents a great danger...*

It is true that sometimes spiritual emergencies are the beginning of an initiation into a deeper aspect of the work (*see my own experience of this on pages 169–170*). When this is the case, they can be seen as 'emergences' rather than 'emergencies'. However, they are unlikely to be easy, and the best advice for all Soul Midwives is to remain grounded and only work within your own boundaries.

Burned-Wing Syndrome

It is particularly important to remember this because we can all get a bit overconfident about our abilities at times. I call this particular problem 'Icarusitis' or 'burned-wing syndrome', after the story of Icarus in Greek mythology. He flew too near the sun and the wax in his wings melted, plunging him back down to Earth. Soul Midwives who are flying too high can experience a subtle and very personal dark night of the soul.

REMEDIES FOR BURNED-WING SYNDROME

- Keep calm and know that these difficulties will pass, even if they feel as if they'll take over your life forever.

- Engage in physical activities such as walking, swimming, yoga, *tai chi* and dancing.

- Go into the countryside and ground yourself. Your body needs fresh air and sunlight in order to rebalance.

- Know that all will be well and your guides will be with you.

- Eat regularly. Frequent small meals help. Foods high in carbs are very grounding. (I always make these dishes for my Soul Midwife courses: cheese and potato pie, vegetable soups, baked pasta dishes, root vegetable curries and stews.)

- Avoid fatty foods (especially meat fat, butter and deep-fried foods), bread, sugar, chocolate, coffee, alcohol, drugs, sweet biscuits, colourings, preservatives, pickles and strong cheeses.

- ✎ Drink plenty of fresh water.

- ✎ Get as much rest as possible. Have a warm bath with Epsom salts before bedtime. Learn some relaxation exercises such as tensing and releasing parts of the body, followed by a meditation before you sleep. Take a cup of chamomile tea to bed with you.

- ✎ At times of difficulty it can help to surrender to the process by saying, 'Not my will, but Thy will' and simply enter a state of humility

BE ALERT AND CAREFUL

When we are working with any form of non-physical state we need to be especially careful. There are certain areas where Soul Midwives can be particularly vulnerable.

Psychopomp Work

Psychopomp work can attract teachers with huge egos; be very cautious about undergoing training without checking the practitioners out first.

I once attended a course on 'letting go' where the facilitator performed several impromptu (dare I say theatrical) exorcisms on some of the participants. Without asking how anyone felt, she powered herself up with a frenzy of chanting. She then made sweeping movements and whooshing noises and used her arms as energetic knives to splice the lost souls from their unknowing hosts. The energy in the room became wounded and anguished as spirits were psychically removed from those they loved.

One of the women in the room had been moaning that her dead mother kept coming shopping with her and bossily advising her on what to buy. Without asking or speaking to the mother, the course leader detached her from her daughter and sent her off into spirit-space, leaving the daughter sobbing because she hadn't had a chance to say goodbye.

Portals

Portals are sacred spaces protected by energetic walls of sound and colour. They are doorways or passages between dimensions which the soul can use to flow back to source. The ancients knew how to create them for the dead to pass through. You'll often find them on ley lines or in vortices, by standing stones, in stone circles and even in churches. In ancient times the energy was powerful at these places and the veils were thin. The dead would have been taken there or buried close by. But As the planet became clogged and dense with stagnant energy, many portals lost their power.

Portals are invisible, but you can feel them if you are sensitive to energies. They have a magnetic suction feeling to them. Some are stronger than others, some are inactive and others are being formed as the Earth's grid changes. Some portals are dark and treacherous, and some are so ecstatic and potent that you can't go near them as their power might distort your energy field.

The key to being able to work with the opportunities of a portal is to attune your vibration to it. In ancient times Soul Midwives worked with sound and crystals to create portals for the souls of the dying to pass through. Some Soul Midwives still do have the natural skills to create portals by intention alone, while others use singing bowls or sound to open them. There are many unconscious dead stuck in the astral realms – souls who are trapped and blanketed from the light – and by opening portals Soul Midwives can help them to move on. They can also use portals to assist friends to pass through the astral realms quickly and consciously.

I use a singing bowl tuned to the note of F sharp. This note is said to have divine qualities, such as the resonance to levitate stones. The great pyramid of Giza is attuned to F sharp. I was also once given a rose quartz and tourmaline portal-maker by a wise woman in southern England's New Forest. I occasionally use it when the veils require a physical key to part them.

You should never attempt to create a portal 'just because you can'. Certainly if you make one, be sure to shut it down again and seal the void.

Soul Loss

Although soul loss is common to shamanic practice, it isn't as well known in other healing modalities. Soul Midwives may be especially vulnerable to it after they have worked and journeyed with a friend beyond the sacred threshold. It happens when we unconsciously leave a part of ourselves behind when we have worked deeply with a friend. This may be due to our particular attachment to them, or perhaps because we didn't honour our return after stepping through the veils.

We are usually protected from this happening just by being mindful of the need to call in all parts of ourselves after working. However, if you are feeling exhausted and generally out of sorts, or attached to a friend who has passed, consult a shamanic practitioner or an experienced Soul Midwife who specializes in soul-retrieval work to retrieve the fragmented part of your soul.

Attachments

Healing can make us very sensitive and open to other energies, especially disincarnate ones who are attracted by the light and come to feed off the energy rush. It is rare, but spirits can attach themselves to us and create problems for our own wellbeing.

Everything is energy, and attachments are conscious beings. Some are aspects of friends we have worked with, others may creep in from past lives and some are even man-made.

COMMON SYMPTOMS OF SPIRIT ATTACHMENT

- ∾ Feeling restless and frustrated.

- ∾ Feeling as if your energy is being drained.

- ∾ Waking up in the early hours and finding it hard to get back to sleep.

- ∾ Sensing or seeing presences.

- ∾ Having sharp pinprick feelings over the legs, hands and arms.

- ∾ Feeling something crawling under your skin.

- ∾ Having unpleasant thoughts in your mind and possibly hearing voices.

- ∾ Feeling despair that doesn't seem to have a cause.

- ∾ Feeling unexplained bursts of anger, sadness or other emotions.

- ∾ Having unexplained fears, phobias or panic attacks.

Some people, especially those who are very sympathetic and of a high vibration, are more susceptible to picking up stray spirits than others. Some environments have greater numbers of discarnate spirits than others. Hospitals tend to have larger numbers of spirits because people die in them. Pubs also tend to attract discarnate spirits because they act as a gathering place for attachments who have been alcoholics and who want the sensation of a drink via a living host.

Thought Forms

Thought forms are also called etheric parasites. They are generated by human thoughts infused with emotion and intent, e.g. the energy that arises from curses, and there are a range of negative thought forms which roam the etheric plane. Like attracts like, and these energetic parasites feed off similar energy to the type that created them. For instance, a parasite created with an angry intention will seek other sources of anger as a host and will induce hateful thoughts in its host to suckle more emotional energy of that type. The negative thought forms generated by one person can induce similar feelings of negativity in another.

People with clairvoyant vision can sometimes see these energy forms – they often look like spiders, crawling ants, microbes and grey-black ink spots. The colours tend to be dull and in muted shades of brown, black, red and orange.

Human 'Spirit' Attachments

These are usually people who have died recently but have not gone to the light, or they have lost their way. They seek out a living person to feed off their energy.

Sometimes, though, a spirit attachment of this type is just an aspect of a person's ego (spirit) that attaches as an energy parasite, and although you can sense it, there is no great substance behind the sensation.

Attachments usually happen when the parasite and living human share a similar vibration. They are usually removed by blocking the attachment from the energy that is feeding them and shifting the vibration rate of the host. The attachments are then sent towards the light with compassion and love.

Consult someone experienced in shamanic work or visit a spirit-release practitioner (*see Resources for details*).

MASTER YOUR SPACE

The best way to care for yourself as a Soul Midwife is to learn to master your space. There's no love like your own, so guard it and strengthen it over time. We live in a world of energy, and releasing negative energy while bringing in positive energy is the most important aspect of our life. This provides true protection from negative energy. This is psychic protection and life-mastery at their finest.

Keep within Safe Boundaries

Be aware of professional boundaries regarding yourself, your patients and their loved ones. In all aspects, you need to take special care to maintain limits, so as not to get burned out and constantly overextend yourself.

Because the basis of our work is a deep offering of one-to-one support, this can make both sides of the partnership vulnerable. In Soul Midwifery, boundaries are not always black and white. Working with a friend for six months before they die is a very different relationship from one with a friend for whom you care only in the last few days of life.

Once a boundary has been broken, it is nearly impossible to restore it. Many of us give our friends or their families our mobile phone numbers. We often receive calls and texts in the middle of the night – even when we're off-duty – but it's very difficult not to respond if you are called. Always be clear about when you are available to work, and when you will not be able to respond.

Physical boundaries can also present difficulties and need to be set on an individual basis. For instance, within some cultures, sitting very close to and touching any part of the body may be viewed as disrespectful. Always ask for permission before you touch anyone, and never assume anything about someone's comfort level or personal space based on culture or age alone.

If you are in a situation where you feel you may be crossing a boundary, ask yourself:

- 'Is what I am offering within my friend's best interests?'

- 'Am I making promises that I might not be able to keep?'

- 'Does my action take away my friend's independence?'

- 'Who is benefitting most from this action?'

- 'Do I stand to gain anything from this action?'

- 'Am I making myself indispensable in order to feel important to the friend or their family?'

Sometimes there is a problem with families becoming over-attached. We can help them with firm kindness and perhaps a referral to a bereavement specialist.

When there seems to be no answer to a particular difficulty, offer it up to the divine and ask for it to be solved for the highest good of all concerned.

Remember to pitch your practice at the level that feels safe and comfortable. Being a Soul Midwife is demanding and heart-precious work and it is important to create safe boundaries of working.

The Four Agreements

Don Miguel Ruiz is a shamanic writer whose inspiring 'four agreements' advice on personal mastery is the backbone of my advice to apprentice Soul Midwives when they begin. I have his advice about always speaking with integrity, never taking anything personally, never making assumptions and always doing your best pinned to the wall above my desk as my own daily guidance.

LIVING IN THE PRESENT

Living in the present is a vital part of self-care. When you truly live in the present you begin to feel everything with a sense of peaceful detachment.

EXERCISE **Focusing on One Simple Thing**

- Begin by noticing every small detail and sensation as you do one simple thing. It could be hearing birdsong outside your kitchen window, getting fresh sheets out of the airing cupboard or opening an old book.

- As you focus on one single sound or impression, you will filter out everything else. Be aware of any sensations, emotions, thoughts and memories that come up. Notice them flowing in and out of your mind without judgement or attachment to them.

- Notice the simple act of slowing down and the pure experience of 'being'.

Breathing exercises and simple yoga or Pilates exercises will also help you to focus on the here and now.

AFFIRMATIONS

Affirmations are statements, either spoken aloud or read silently, that set an intention. You have seen examples of them throughout this book. Once you have made an affirmation and internalized it, it becomes real on the subtle levels.

Affirming that you have let go of and been released from a contract with a friend will help to keep your energy clear and dissolve any obligations to them.

EXERCISE Letting It Go

'If I look after someone who is dying, will I be affected by their pain and suffering?' Apprentice Soul Midwives often ask this question and here is the answer: breathe in the suffering, surround it with light, then breathe it out again... let it go.

- Lie down flat with your arms at your sides.

- Close your eyes and take 15 deep breaths.

- When you feel ready, repeat the words 'let' and 'go', either silently to yourself or out loud. Breathing in, say 'let' and breathing out, say 'go'.

- Repeat this.

You may find that your mind tries to distract you with chattering thoughts, but gently bring your attention back to saying 'let' and 'go'.

A Prayer of Affirmation for Soul Midwives

In this work I am totally aligned with light, love, truth and resonance with human consciousness. I offer my care and time.

It is my intention to create a state of grace within my own heart which may illuminate a path for others.

I am aware that we each as divine beings follow our own path, and I offer to support and honour those I care for to enable them to deepen their own experience of the divine.

I recognize that the upheaval and change that transition presents are necessary for the ripening of the soul, and this is a sacred opportunity to integrate the consciousness of life and reconnect with source.

I thank you, spirit, for your presence in my consciousness and your inspiration in my service as a Soul Midwife. And so it is.

Amen

SUMMARY

- Soul Midwives need to take good care of themselves in order to care for others.

- Cleansing and protecting our own energy fields are important aspects of spiritual hygiene.

- Working with deep empathy and sympathy requires us to be masters of our own psyche.

- Soul work is demanding. We need to know how to dissolve energy connections with our friends and revitalize ourselves.

- We need to establish safe boundaries for our own wellbeing.

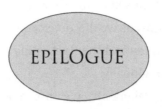

SOUL MIDWIFERY AND THE WIDER PICTURE

'If you send forth love to others, you will receive in return the reflection of that love: and you will shine a light that will brighten the darkness of the time we live in — whether it is in the sickroom of a dying patient, on the corner of a ghetto in Harlem, or in your own home.'
ELISABETH KÜBLER-ROSS

So far in this handbook we have looked at the primary role of the Soul Midwife at the bedside of the dying person. We have learned how to accompany someone from the point of diagnosis through the dying process and the metamorphosis of transition into the great beyond.

Just for a moment, though, imagine how this huge event that affects every individual soul reflects the wider picture of our place within the universe.

Just as there are Soul Midwives for the dying, so there are also planetary Soul Midwives, whose work is to hold and anchor new energies and soothe the birth pangs of a new paradigm. These Soul

Midwives are the lightworkers who are helping the planet as she raises her levels of consciousness.

As human beings, we are the cells of the living body of this planet, and are therefore sharing in the birth of this expanded consciousness. And just as we are composed of the four elements – Earth, Water, Fire and Air – which withdraw as we die, or ascend, so, as the planet ascends, the same dynamic unfolds and the fluctuating energies experienced by the dying are mirrored globally.

As we release the elements, we lose our energetic equilibrium. We wobble, lose our way and experience the realms of chaos. When this happens, we are invariably challenged by our shadow side rising from our deep subconscious. Negative patterns we thought we had conquered may suddenly jump out of the dark and surprise us. Unless we have worked with them, ripened our souls (by pushing through our comfort zones) and developed our awareness and compassion, we'll be in for a bumpy ride. So, too, the elemental transitions of ascension cause imbalance in the world around us.

We are spiritual beings living in human bodies. The same applies to the planet. She, too, is spiritual, yet physical in her being, with her mountains, valleys, oceans and continents. What are the effects as she rebalances her energy systems and accelerates her frequencies, retuning to a higher note?

The extreme events caused by climate change in recent years – earthquakes, droughts, fires, floods, storms and tsunamis – are signs of the Earth's changes. On the human level, there has been increasing social unrest, the toppling of major financial and political institutions and a lack of faith and confidence in government and organized religion by the mass population. These huge shifts in stability on a global scale mirror the inner feelings experienced by a dying person swept up by energetic imbalances.

The three distinct psycho-spiritual phases of the dying process – chaos, surrender and transcendence – are also mirrored by the planet.

Chaos manifests both physically – weather, volcanoes, eruptions, crises, health epidemics – and in feelings of fear and duality. We may suffer 'total pain' – a palliative care term for the merging of physical, psychic and emotional pain.

COMMON ASCENSION/TRANSITION SYMPTOMS

- We can feel off-balance and disorientated.

- Our vision may not seem as good, although this can fluctuate from day to day (sometimes we feel pressure behind the eyes).

- Our body may retain fluid and/or feel bloated.

- Our back (spine) may feel sore, stiff and/or out of alignment.

- Our heart may pound and we may experience thudding palpitations.

- There may be strange ringing in our ears.

Surrender comes as global communities begin to think outside the box and reject old fear-based regimes. This is the tipping point when things have to change in order to evolve. We may feel extreme disconnection from the norm, as everything we grasp slips through our fingers and, like Alice in Wonderland, we tumble down a hole into a strange new world.

Transcendence finally comes after the struggle, as love and heart wisdom replace power struggles and fear-based dogma. When your heart has opened, it is no longer possible to treat other people unkindly and the whole world changes.

Shamanic and esoteric teachings have always shown that in order to be initiated into something greater we have to 'die to the old', and also that our death carries all the potential required for huge leaps of soul growth and ascension.

In both living and dying we make our choices to feed our soul's requirements for evolution. These opportunities for soul growth offer us many rich gifts, lessons and challenges. They manifest all our life until we reach a soul state where shifting our vibration to a higher level becomes the main goal.

This is the great key to seeing the connection between the ascension of the planet and the transition of human consciousness after death.

THE JOURNEY AHEAD

Who am I? Why am I here? Where did I come from? What did I learn? Where am I going? In times of great transition, both on an individual and a global level, people ask the big questions. Yet these are just preparation for the dying/transition/ascension process...

We can work with these ideas and develop them into a 'thinking map' for the journey ahead, asking ourselves:

- 'What do I need to learn?'

- 'What am I ready to release and give up?'

- 'How can I consciously embrace the changes and potential of the current moment?'

- 'How can I embrace these changes as an experience for soul growth?'

Depending on our level of consciousness, we either regain our balance by detaching, releasing and replacing fear with love, or we enter the dark night of the soul – an experience that forces us to go with the flow – before the exquisite bliss of transcendence eventually embraces us.

EXERCISE Staying Calm through Planetary Transition

- Stabilize your energy field three times a day. To do this, find a quiet moment to imagine a giant hook pulling from your feet down to the core of the Earth. Imagine another hooking you up to the highest point in the heavens. Feel the strength in being held by these two points, and feel your energy field being equally distributed between these two hooks.

- Relax and stay calm – take time out, use your answerphone instead of taking calls, only check your e-mails once a day.

- When you are challenged by something, think from the heart and centre yourself.

- Don't take things personally.

- Practise being the still centre of the storm by breathing steadily and keeping a calm focus.

- Don't be attached to outcomes.

- Drink plenty of water and eat fresh food.

- If you go into an energy storm and feel depleted, rest, meditate and eat carbohydrates to ground yourself.

- Take regular exercise.

- Breathe calmly and consciously.

- Use fragonia and palo santo essential oils to balance your energy field.

EASING INTO ASCENSION

This is an opportunity to understand the deepest levels of ourselves as humans, whilst inviting spirit to guide us at every moment. In doing this, we stay connected to our pure essence rather than the personality or ego.

Despite the chaos, ascension and transition should be a gentle journey of discovery, leading us into a greater level of awareness, unity and joy.

Globally, things may appear to be on the brink as we all start to think and act outside the box, but this is just the illusion of change and flux. Like the dying person facing infinity, we have now all reached the tipping point of surrender. We are only a step away from transcendence in planetary and soul time. We can now allow the power of the divine source to gently move us towards a higher vibration.

Collectively, we are stepping across the sacred threshold and into the light.

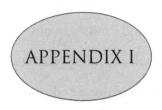

APPENDIX I

GETTING STARTED

You can start work as a Soul Midwife in several ways. If you already work in the caring or medical professions, you may be able to undertake Soul Midwife training (*see pages 259–264*) and incorporate what you have learned into your current working practice. This will also be the case if you are an established alternative therapist.

If you do not have a background in therapy, however, you should consider undertaking training in energy work (such as Reiki), counselling, celebrancy or vigiling in addition to your Soul Midwife training.

Gaining Experience

Once you have completed your training, however you decide to use your Soul Midwifery skills you must volunteer at a local hospice or care home and build up your practical experience. The real work cannot be done until you have spent many hours sitting at the bedsides of the dying.

Once you are confident that you have the experience to work as a Soul Midwife, start slowly. Gain confidence by taking small steps like offering death-planning sessions, holding 'Let's talk about death' coffee mornings and giving talks to local groups.

Advertising

You may also want to advertise your services. Here are some ideas:

- Print business cards and hand them out.

- Link with professionals providing related services in your area.

- Write articles for the local press and community magazines and contact your local radio station.

- Put flyers in local healthfood shops, new age shops and complementary medicine clinics.

You should also consider setting up a website, as most people looking for a Soul Midwife search the internet. There are many firms offering website design packages quite cheaply.

It's worth noting that clients respond better to a web presence when they can feel they are connecting with a real person. They want a midwife with integrity, one who comes from the heart. So keep your biographical details short, but include how long you have been a practising Soul Midwife, why you do it and what inspired you to do the work.

A website is also useful for providing free advice, inspiration and links to other sites. Be clear about your charging structure, to avoid confusion later on.

Insurance

Please note that you are likely to need insurance and criminal record checks to work as a Soul Midwife. In the UK you will need professional indemnity insurance and a Disclosure and Barring Service (DBS) check. Please check the appropriate regulations for your local area.

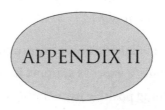

APPENDIX II

REFLECTIONS AND RECORDS

Reflections

After each session with a friend, it is important to assess their changing needs and aspirations and assess whether you are helping them to fulfil them. For example, after each interaction with a friend you could ask yourself, 'Did I...':

- actively listen to my friend without judgement?

- help my friend identify and prioritize their goals for the dying experience *they* wish to achieve?

- demonstrate a belief in my friend's existing strengths and resources in relation to the pursuit of their expectations?

- identify examples from my own life experience (or from those of other dying friends) which can inspire and validate their hopes?

- pay particular attention to the importance of thoughts/inspirations which take my friend out of their 'sick role' and enable them to actively contribute to the lives of others?

- identify non-holistic resources – friends, contacts and organizations – relevant to the achievement of their goals?

- discuss what they needed in terms of therapeutic assistance?

- convey an attitude of respect for my friend and a desire for an equal partnership in our work?

- accept that the immediate future is uncertain and setbacks will happen, but continue to express support for my friend in achieving goals and maintaining positive expectations?

Records

Keep detailed written records of each session. This will help you to focus on any subtle changes and act as a reminder of the work you have done with your friend.

In the UK, all personal information must be kept in accordance with the Data Protection Act 1998:

- You must obtain permission from your friend to keep any personal information.

- The information must be limited to your needs only and kept only as long as is needed.

- You must maintain confidentiality and not pass on any information.

- All personal information must be secure: kept in a locked filing cabinet or computerized with a password.

Note that you may need to register with the Data Protection Registrar if you intend to keep information about your friends on a computer – it is easier to keep manual notes.

You will need to check out specific legal requirements in your country for data protection, as this varies across the globe.

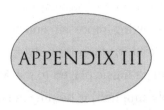

A SAMPLE END-OF-LIFE PLAN

Jane Fryer

Age 57; Condition: Lung cancer

These are the people who are most important in my life:

- John, my husband

- Joan, my mother (now 88 and frail, living in Freelands Residential Home, West Heath)

- Kate, my daughter, who lives in London, mother of my grandchildren: Lizzie (7) and Caleb (10)

My doctor is Dr Prior, West Field Health Centre, West Heath (but I don't get on with him very well and always book to see Dr Hurst).

I would like to die at home (possibly in the garden if it is a nice day), with my husband and children around and about. I would like to be able to hear normal family life going on around me.

People I do not want to have with me are my sister and her husband, from whom I am estranged.

Holistic treatments I find enjoyable and helpful are meditation, massage and music (I do not like having my feet touched).

Things I am frightened of: I would like to learn some breathing exercises while I am still well, as I am frightened of not being able to catch my breath towards the end. I saw my dad really suffering when he died and this has left a lasting impression on me.

I would like to be told if/when I am dying, and in my last hours I would like some favourite music played to me. My Soul Midwife (Sarah Hughes; contact details supplied) is helping me to make a CD up of this music and I will have it in my bedroom.

When I have died I would like to be left peacefully for three days if possible before being removed for burial. (My Soul Midwife and my husband have already arranged this with the undertaker.)

I would like to be buried in my favourite red flannel nightdress and wrapped in the pink quilt that I made and have stored in the blanket box at the end of my bed.

When I am feeling well I like to see my family and friends, including my best friend, Pat, who lives in Truro. I would like visits to be limited to an hour or so, as I get tired, but some visitors don't appear to notice. I probably need visits to be discreetly timed by someone to check that they don't overrun.

On bad days, when I am not feeling well, I just like to be quiet. I don't want to talk but I love to have very quiet company and someone to hold my hand.

I like to feel clean and to have my hair brushed and my nails looking nice.

I like to have my two cats sleeping with me.

I like watching funny DVDs (I have Mr Bean and Monty Python DVDs for down days).

I would like to have pictures of my friends and favourite places in Cornwall in my room as I am dying, and also a CD with sounds of the sea and seagulls in the background.

I would not like to be resuscitated or given antibiotics for infections if I am taken into hospital.

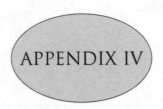

APPENDIX IV

REQUIREMENTS AT THE TIME OF DEATH

Legal Requirements

Always make a note of the time of death. In the UK, the death must be certified and registered and the body must be disposed of in accordance with the Births and Deaths Registration Act 1926.

There may well be different legal requirements locally, depending on which country or state you live in. Be sure to check out your legal position.

The Requirements of Different Faiths

Here is a quick guide to the requirements of different faiths at the time of death:

Buddhist

Specific prayers and chants may be recited and the Bardo practice may be offered for 49 days after death. The body should be left undisturbed for three days following death.

Christian

It is customary to recite the Lord's Prayer at the time of death.

Hindu

If possible, a Hindu should die lying on the floor, so they have contact with the Earth. Touching the corpse is frowned upon, other than by certain relatives.

Islamic

The body should be buried within 24 hours of death. Family members or friends will perform the ritual washing. Females wash females and males wash males.

Jewish

Notify the Chevra Kadisha, the organization that will prepare the body for burial and help make the funeral arrangements. Jewish burials are usually held within 24 hours of death.

❧ GLOSSARY ❧

Affirmation: an expression of intent that is spoken out loud or written down to bring positive change to a situation.

Algor mortis: cooling of the body after death.

Anointing: smearing or rubbing the body with oil to signify a blessing or a symbol of intent; useful in releasing any troubles that are making peaceful transition difficult.

Aromatherapy: the inhalation and application to the body of oils derived from plants to bring both inner and outer balance and well-being. Within Soul Midwifery essential oils may be used to alter the energy of the lightbody.

Aura: an electromagnetic field surrounding the human body. People with enhanced psychic ability are able to see the movement, shape and varied colours of the aura.

Ayurvedic medicine: a 3,000–5,000-year-old system of healthcare practised in India. The fundamental belief in the Ayurvedic system is that everything living in the universe is composed of *prana* (life force). Treatment focuses on balancing the four elements or the *doshas*: *vatha* (elements of mostly Water and Earth), *pitta* (elements of Fire and some Water) and *kapha* (elements of Air and Space).

Brain death: a condition that results when the brain ceases to be conscious and the body operates only as a result of mechanical assistance. There are no brainwaves, movements or responses to stimuli.

Chakras: the major vortices of energy which act as the junction points between mind and matter, allowing us to draw in life-force energy to fuel our body. A chakra is shaped like a funnel and acts like one, directing energy into the body. When the chakras are blocked or closed, our energy intake is diminished and we start to lose our ability to function at an optimal level.

Clairvoyance: the gift of second sight. People who are clairvoyant are able to perceive or intuit information by seeing auras, colours, images or symbols via their third eye. They may also be clairaudient (able to pick up information via inner hearing) or clairsentient (able to gain information through feeling or sensory experience).

Comfort care: treatment whose focus is to improve the quality of life through pain management and relief from psychological, emotional and spiritual stress.

Complementary therapies: holistic treatments used alongside mainstream medicine. Examples include art therapy, music therapy, massage and acupuncture.

Death-rattle: the noise made by a dying person as the breath passes through mucus when the cough reflex is lost.

Egyptian *Book of the Dead*: a set of 200 spells and prayers to assist a dead person on their trip to the next world. It was written on papyrus before 1400 BCE.

Energy blocks: in addition to our physical body we have an energy body, which can become blocked for many reasons, such as stress and anxiety, physical injuries, shock and emotional upset. If these blockages are not cleared, they can manifest as physical, mental or emotional illness. Healers are able to channel energies through their hands that can help to release blockages and encourage the body's own natural healing process to take place.

Energy fields: fields of energy holding a vibration that is created when several people resonate and work with the same intention.

Energy healing: *see vibrational healing.*

Flower/floral waters: *see hydrolats.*

Hathors: ascended masters working specifically with the energy fields of sound and love to transmute fear and duality in individuals undergoing transition, and also in global systems and structures.

Healing touch: touch that balances and aligns the body's energy system. It increases relaxation and helps to decrease the stress response, promoting positive changes in attitudes, behaviour, thoughts and emotions. When there is balance in body, mind and spirit, the body will heal itself naturally. Healing touch facilitates this process by realigning the energy flow, thus reactivating the mind, body, spirit connection and eliminating blockages.

Herbal medicine: medicine that harnesses the healing constituents of specific plants (found in their leaves, stalks, roots, seeds and petals).

Hospice: a form of palliative care in which the main focus is on comfort rather than cure. Generally, people in hospice care have elected to forego curative treatments and often enrol when they have a life expectancy of less than six months. In the US, hospice care often takes place in a patient's home.

Hydrolat/hydrosol: a by-product of the distillation process used in obtaining pure essential oils. Also known as flower or floral water.

Hydrosol: *see hydrolat.*

Lament: a traditional song for the dying.

Last offices: the services provided by a nurse shortly after death, including washing and preparing the body for the undertaker.

Lightbody: the sum of a person's energetic layers, from the densest physical body to the subtlest spiritual body.

Myrrhophores: an esoteric fellowship of women adepts, high initiates and priestly scientists who work with the mysteries of consciousness and vibrationary fields.

Palliative care: *see comfort care.*

Past lives: lives we have had prior to the present one.

Portals: vortices and conduits, either already existing or created through intention, through which energy and consciousness can travel between dimensions.

Shaman: a person with the ability to go beyond normally perceived reality to connect with other realms of consciousness. The shaman directs their intent (the basis of any transformation) to manifest change, empowerment and healing. Shamanic consciousness consistently uses connections with the Earth, spirit animals and guides.

Singing bowls/temple bells: ritual instruments, traditionally made from seven different metals, which can be struck or played

Soul: the eternal aspect of who we are, which continues to evolve after each incarnation. It is a fragment of our divine connection with source.

Soul Midwives: non-medical companions to the dying who offer spiritual and holistic support, honouring death as a sacred, tranquil and dignified experience. Soul Midwives draw on traditional skills to ease the passage of the dying, and their services can be provided in a home, hospital or a hospice setting. Advanced Soul Midwives are also technicians of consciousness working with transition at all levels.

Soul wounds: the fundamental wounds in our psyche, caused by our separation from the divine/source. Typically, they manifest as feelings of abandonment, lack of self-worth and fear. We may also carry cultural soul wounds and karmic soul wounds from past lives.

Sound bath: a massage with sound given to friends at the bedside. It is usually created with percussive instruments – singing bowls, finger cymbals, chimes, rain sticks and crystal sound bowls – but also harps and sounding bowls.

Spirit: the ego-based aspect of our identity which leaves the body at death and gradually disappears.

Temple bells: *see singing bowls.*

Terminal agitation: a common symptom at the end of life; may include the inability to relax, picking at clothing or sheets, confusion and agitation, and trying to climb out of bed.

Thanatology: the study of the social and psychological aspects of death and dying, practised by thanatologists.

Transition: Soul Midwife term to describe the process of dying, or moving from one level of consciousness to another.

Unconditional love: loving from the heart without judgement or the expectation of outcome.

Vibrational/energy healing: When two things vibrate at different frequencies, the law of resonance requires that the lower frequency comes up or the upper frequency goes down, or that they meet in the middle. Vibrational/energy healers learn to hold a high vibration in their hands so that the friend receiving the healing will eventually match that vibration.

Vibrational remedies: remedies, usually taken internally or rubbed on the skin or added to bathwater, which help to rebalance the body's etheric electrical system. In these times we are all being required to release the old fears that are blocking our spiritual progress. Vibrational remedies such as flower essences and gem elixirs work quickly, gently and powerfully to help us do this.

Visualization: using the imagination to create images/scenarios that can be used for healing and relaxation.

❧ RECOMMENDED READING ❧

Death and Dying

Phyllida Anam-Aire, *The Celtic Book of Dying*, Findhorn Press, 2005

Patricia Davis, *Aromatherapy: An A–Z*, The C. W. Daniel Company, 1988

Peter and Elizabeth Fenwick, *The Art of Dying*, Continuum, 2010

Graceful Exits: How Great Beings Die, ed. Sushila Blackman, Shambhala Press, 2005

Michael Kearney, *A Place of Healing*, Spring Journal Books, 2009

Betty Kovacs, *The Miracle of Death*, Kamalak, 2003

Elisabeth Kübler-Ross, *On Death and Dying*, Routledge, 1970

Anita Moorjani, *Dying to Be Me*, Hay House, 2011

Sherwin B. Nuland, MD, *How We Die*, Chatto & Windus, 1993

Sam Parnia, *What Happens When We Die?*, Hay House, 2005

Richard Reoch, *Dying Well*, Gaia, 1997

Sogyal Rinpoche, *The Tibetan Book of Living and Dying*, Rider, 1992

Mary Anne Saunders, *Nearing Death Awareness*, JKP Books, 2007

Kathleen Dowling Singh, *The Grace in Dying*, Newleaf, 1999

Starhawk, *The Pagan Book of Living and Dying*, HarperSanFrancisco, 1997

The Tibetan Book of the Dead, ed. Robert A. F. Thurman, The Aquarian Press, 1994

Healing and Energy Medicine

Harriet Beinfield and Efrem Korngold, *Between Heaven and Earth: A Guide to Chinese Medicine*, Ballantine Books, 1991

Barbara Brennan, *Hands of Light*, Bantam Books, 1988

Donna Eden, *Energy Medicine*, Tarcher/Putnam, 1998

Gill Edwards, *Living Magically*, Piatkus Books, 1991

—, *Conscious Medicine*, Piatkus Books, 2010

Caroline Myss, *Anatomy of the Spirit*, Bantam Books, 1997

Norman Shealy and Dawson Church, *Soul Medicine*, Elite Books, 2006

Rupert Sheldrake, *The Presence of the Past: Morphic Resonance and the Habits of Nature*, HarperCollins, 1988

Herbs/Oils/Flower Essences

Dr Bruce Berkowsky, *Essential Oils and the Cancer Miasm*, Joseph Ben Hil-Meyer Research Press, 2000

Clare Harvey, *The New Encyclopedia of Flower Remedies*, Watkins, 2007

Eliseo Torres and Timothy L. Sawyer, *Healing with Herbs and Rituals: A Mexican Tradition*, University of New Mexico Press, 2006

George Vithoulkas, *The Science of Homeopathy*, Grove Press, 1980

Elizabeth M. Williamson, *Potter's Herbal Cyclopedia*, The C. W. Daniel Company, 2003

Music
Leslie Bunt, *Music Therapy*, Routledge, 1994

Carol A. Bush, *Healing Imagery and Music*, Rudra Press, 1995

Jonathan Goldman, *Healing Sounds*, Healing Arts Press, 1992

Susan Elizabeth Hale, *Sacred Space, Sacred Sound*, Quest Books, 2007

Eva Rudy Jansen, *Singing Bowls*, Binkey Kok Publications, 1990

Psychic Protection
William Bloom, *Feeling Safe*, Piatkus Books, 2002

Judy Hall, *Good Vibrations*, Flying Horse Books, 2008

Terry and Natalia O'Sullivan, *Soul Rescuers*, Thorsons, 1999

Soul/Dying
Dolores Cannon, *Between Death and Life*, Gateway, 1993

James Hillman, *Suicide and the Soul*, Spring Publications, 1965

—, *The Soul's Code*, Bantam Books, 1996

Barry Long, *Behind Life and Death*, Barry Long Books, 2008

Kristin Madden, *The Shamanic Guide to Death and Dying*, Spilled Candy Books, 1999

Starhawk, *The Spiral Dance*, Harper and Row, 1979

Spirituality/Ritual/Shamanism

Dolores Ashcroft-Nowicki, *The New Book of the Dead*, The Aquarian Press, 1992

Deepak Chopra, *The Book of Secrets*, Rider, 2004

Mircea Eliade, *Shamanisn: Archaic Techniques of Ecstasy*, Arkana, 1989

Helen Greaves, *Testimony of Light*, Rider, 1969

Stephen Levine, *Healing into Life and Death*, Anchor Press, 1987

Raymond J. Moody, *Life After Life*, Bantam Books, 1975

Robert Moss, *Dreamgates: An Explorer's Guide to the Worlds of Soul, Imagination, and Life Beyond Death*, Three Rivers Press, 1998

Michael Newton, *Journey of Souls*, Llewellyn Publications, 2003

Don Miguel Ruiz, *The Four Agreements*, Amber Allen Publishing, 1997

Eckhart Tolle, *The Power of Now*, New World Library, 1999

Eliseo Torres, *Curandero: A Life in Mexican Folk Healing*, University of New Mexico Press, 2005

Vigiling and Prayer

Megory Anderson, *Sacred Dying*, Marlowe and Company, 2001

Tess Ward, *The Celtic Wheel of the Year*, O Books, 2007

❧ RESOURCES ❧

The Soul Midwives' Tool Kit

The following items are available via the Soul Midwives' School (www.soulmidwives.co.uk):

- *Essential oils:* A comprehensive range of oils specifically for use in Soul Midwifery. Many of the oils that Soul Midwives use are unusual and hard to source. The school stocks a selection of the most sacred and useful oils, including anointing oils for assisting transition.

- *Prayer beads:* These beautiful prayer beads are designed for Soul Midwives or their friends. They loop over your index finger and sit in the palm of your hand. You then say a prayer while holding each bead. The beads are smooth and tactile and are designed to bring a sense of peace, love and grounding. Different beads and prayers are available; for example, to re-energize a Soul Midwife after working with a friend or to bring a friend comfort during pain, or when experiencing the Water stage.

- *Vibrational remedies:* Flower and tree essences, including elemental remedies (autumn wind, lightning, snowflake, etc.), to support the four stages of element withdrawal.

- *Vigiling candles:* These handcrafted candles, in a variety of colours, are infused with sacred oils for use in vigiling and celebrancy.

Other Suppliers

- *Crystal bowls:* www.enterprise-q.co.uk

- *Candles and Chalice Well (Glastonbury) water for blessings and rituals:* www.chalicewell.org.uk

- *Essential oils:* materiaaromatica.com

- *Harps/lyres/a large range of other instruments:* www.soundtravels.co.uk

- *Mohair blankets:* Bronte at Home: brontebydesign.co.uk

- *Singing bowls:* Frank Perry: frankperry.co.uk

- *Soap made from the holy water at Lourdes:* www.immaculatewaters.com

- *Sounding bowls:* www.soundingbowls.com

- *Tuning forks:* www.biosonics.com

- *Wraps, quilts and rainbow curtains:* hazelrowntreecounselling

Funerals

For contemporary funeral directors and courses in the UK, see:

- www.goodfuneralguide.co.uk

- *Green Fuse:* greenfuse.co.uk (Jane Morrell and Simon Smith). Their other website is also recommended: www.weneedtotalkaboutthefuneral.com.

- *Elizabeth Way Family Funeral Service:* elizabeth-way.co.uk (Gail Dyson)

Coffin suppliers:

- *Felt shrouds and woollen coffins:* www.yulisomme.co.uk

- *Willow coffins:* www.musgrovewillowcoffins.co.uk

Memory Work

- You can use storylane.com or storycorps.org to record memories and family stories, or thankingofyou.com to post a story of gratitude in written or videotaped form.

- Use voicequilt.com to invite family and friends to record messages on a toll-free voice-message system – just like leaving messages on an answering machine. Your friend can then listen to the messages online.

- If your friend is finding it difficult to dial phone numbers, you could recommend FotoDialer (see photodialing.com). It attaches to an existing phone, but instead of dialing numbers you press a picture of a loved one: it's a combination of photo album and speed dial.

- Check out bagsoflove.co.uk for different ways to use family photos to create gifts.

Music

Below is a list of some recorded music you may consider using at the bedside:

- Lynn Morrison, *Cave of Gold*

- Arvo Pärt, *Litany*

- The chants of the Céile Dé (*Fonn*); see ceilede.co.uk

- Rosemary Duxbury, *Streams*, *Thread of Gold* and *On Wings of Light*

- Annie Lennox, 'Into the West', *The Return of the King* soundtrack

Toning and chakra CDs:

- Jonathan Goldman and Crystal Tones, *Crystal Bowls Chakra Chants*

- Jonathan Goldman, *Healing Sounds Instructional* (toning and overtoning)

You might also like to look at the work of:

- Michael Chamberlain, who offers sound healing events and workshops: www.soundsalive.org

- Elizabeth Hornby, a young composer/pianist who is producing some CDs for Soul Midwives to use at the bedside: www.elizabethpiano.tictail.com

- music thanatologist and harpist Abigail Robinson: www.sacred-sound.co.uk

Reiki

If you wish to study Reiki, find a recommended Reiki Master and talk about being attuned to Reiki I (the self-healing level). (There are lots of Soul Midwife Reiki Masters, so please feel free to ask the Soul Midwives' School if there are any in your area who can attune you.) It is important that you feel comfortable and relaxed with your potential Reiki Master, as this will be an ongoing relationship.

Follow Reiki I with Reiki II (healing others, using Reiki symbols and distance healing). There is also a third level for more advanced practitioners and a teaching level (Master training).

It is always useful to consider obtaining an 'anatomy and physiology' qualification before practising any form of alternative therapy. However, according to the UK Reiki Federation, it is not compulsory for practitioners to have an A&P qualification in order to practise Reiki and to obtain insurance (although you should check with individual insurers). The UK Reiki Federation: www.reikifed.co.uk.

Spiritual Help

The Spirit Release Forum, a meeting place for those interested in exploring spirit release issues, offers a list of qualified spirit release practitioners: www.spiritrelease.org

Spiritual Crisis Network offers an e-mail support service providing general information on spiritual crisis and facilitates a UK national network of local groups of people with experience, interest or involvement in spiritual crisis: www.spiritualcrisisnetwork.org.uk

Useful Websites

International Organizations

Death Cafés
At death cafés, people come together in a relaxed and safe setting to discuss death, drink tea and eat delicious cakes! www.deathcafé.com

The Association for Comprehensive Energy Psychology
www.energypsych.org

The International Academy for Interfaith Studies
interfaithacademy.org

The International Society for Complementary Medicine Research
An international professional, multidisciplinary, non-profit scientific organization devoted to fostering complementary and integrative medicine research: www.iscmr.org

Australia

The Complementary Medicine Association Australia
cma.asn.au

Canada

The Canadian Association for Integrative and Energy Therapies
(CAIET)
www.caiet.org

The Spirituality in Health-Care Network
www.spiritualityinhealthcare.net

The United Kingdom

The Association of Professional Music Therapists
www.apmt.org

Balens
Offers professional indemnity cover for Soul Midwives:
www.balens.co.uk

Breathwork
For breathing techniques: www.holotropic.com

The British Complementary Medicine Association
www.bcma.co.uk

The British Holistic Medical Association
www.bhma.org

The British Society for Music Therapy
www.bsmt.org

Cancer Research UK
Information and support for cancer: http://www.cancerresearchuk.org

The Centre for Death and Society (CDAS)
The UK's only centre devoted to the study and research of the social aspects of death, dying and bereavement: www.bath.ac.uk

The Complementary and Alternative Medicines in Cancer Consortium
www.cam-cancer.org

Dying Matters
A national organization/platform relating to all aspects of death and dying: www.dyingmatters.org

Elemental Withdrawal
There is a powerful meditation relating to the elemental stages and dissolution of the body at death by Joan Halifax Roshi: www.upaya.org/roshi/dox/dissolution.pdf. Her website is also worth a visit: upaya.org/roshi

The Healing Trust
The new working name for the National Federation of Spiritual Healers Charitable Trust. Pan-denominational organization for spiritual healers: www.thehealingtrust.org.uk

Help the Hospices
The leading charity supporting hospice care throughout the UK: www.helpthehospices.org.uk

Horizon Research Foundation
An independent charitable organization supporting scientific research and understanding into the state of the human mind at the end of life: www.horizonresearch.org

The Institute for Complementary and Natural Medicine
www.icnm.org.uk

The International Association for Near-Death Studies
www.iands.org

Final Fling
An informative website looking at death and dying and everything surrounding it: www.finalfling.com

The Martinsey Isle Trust
A not-for-profit organization involved in a variety of work connected to death and dying: www.marrtinsey.org.uk

Medicdirect
www.medicdirect.co.uk/alt_medicines

The National Association of Complementary Therapists in Hospice and Palliative Care
www.nacthpc.org.uk

The Natural Death Centre
Provides a helpline and loads of advice on the choices relating to funerals and burials: naturaldeath.org.uk

OneSpirit Interfaith Foundation
www.interfaithfoundation.org

Antonia Rolls
A Soul Midwife who tours the UK with 'A Graceful Death' exhibition:
www.agracefuldeath.blogspot.co.uk

Therapy Directory
www.therapy-directory.org.uk

The Transitus Network
A growing group of people working in a way that honours all aspects of life that are involved with the sacred process of dying:
www.transitus.co.uk

The United States of America

The Chalice of Repose Project
A music therapy project within hospices in the USA:

www.chaliceofrepose.org

MD Anderson Cancer Center's Complementary/Integrative Medicine Education Resources
Information about complementary therapies in cancer care:
www.mdanderson.org/departments/CIMER/

The Memorial Sloan-Kettering Cancer Center: Integrative Medicine Service
A leading cancer hospital and research centre in New York. They have a helpful database on herbs and botanical products.
www.mskcc.org/mskcc

The Sacred Dying Foundation
Offers spiritual care: www.sacreddying.org

The US National Cancer Institute's National Center for Complementary and Alternative Medicine (NCCAM)
NCCAM is an American government-funded institution that supports scientific research into complementary and alternative therapies:
http://nccam.nih.gov

The US National Institute of Health Office of Cancer Complementary and Alternative Medicine
The cancer-specific section of the US National Institute of Health:
www.cancer.gov/cancertopics/cam

The US National Library of Medicine and the National Institutes of Health
This US site has information about complementary and alternative therapies. It provides detailed information about herbs and supplements, as well as the latest news on various therapies: www.nlm.nih.gov/medlineplus/complementaryandalternativemedicine.html

THE SOUL MIDWIVES' SCHOOL

After so many years of working with the dying, teaching and passing on my knowledge of Soul Midwifery is a passion.

In the beginning, ten years ago, I was coaxed into offering afternoon sessions in my home by people who wanted to learn how to sit with their own loved ones. It wasn't that I had all the answers – far from it – but by then I did have experience, insights and certainly enthusiasm. If I didn't know the answers to all the extraordinary questions that came up, I would say so and try to find someone who did.

Eventually, as word spread, I'd find myself talking to groups of palliative care professionals. At first I felt nervous about explaining my methods – they seemed so simple and homespun. I thought I'd be shot down and laughed at, challenged and heckled for my audacity, but I wasn't. Instead I received more invitations to speak.

People were hungry for information about dying, but also for an opportunity to share deep personal experiences. I noticed that when healthcare workers undertook the gentle therapies, they used them to heal themselves and open up conversations with each other. In one group two medical social workers who worked with dying children talked of the 'spirit children' who visited them to say hello and to pass on messages to their parents. A GP confided that she knew immediately if her patients were dying, as she picked up 'information' as they walked into her surgery. Another confided to the group that his dead patients sometimes came back to talk to him.

Over the years many doctors and nurses have come on my courses and expressed relief at being able to share their unusual experiences. Healthcare professionals see so much pain and suffering on a daily basis and have no outlets for sharing. They are often exhausted, run down and running on dry.

On the courses, people wanted to share ideas about the nature of death, the soul and the life beyond. As they weren't able to have these conversations at work, they found the workshops useful as a safe place in which to express their ideas and feelings.

I began by teaching very simple things, such as how to talk to someone who has just learned that they are terminally ill. I wanted to show that we can explain that they have choices about what will happen to them, what sort of therapies might help and when to use them. This collection of tips and techniques, known as the Gentle Dying method, gradually evolved into the much deeper practice of Soul Midwifery.

When I look back at the early days of running courses, I'm astonished that people came and listened and believed in me. I was initially very cautious about how much esoteric information I offered, but over time the limits have stretched beyond my expectations and people have expanded their knowledge base. This has helped me grow to teach what is now a very eclectic syllabus!

I started to be invited to national conferences to talk about my work. I also lectured in hospitals, hospices and universities all over the UK and beyond. People who read my books began to visit me, and now I have trained Soul Midwives across the world.

It's important to me that the courses are intimate and loving. Most of them are still held in my home beside the fire. I mix the oils and make the essences we work with and I cook and serve the food. Hospitality and sharing homeliness are such important ways of showing how we can give love and tenderness to others at the end of life.

Many people who come on the courses work in institutions where every aspect of their work and training is audited, quality controlled, tick-boxed and delivered with health and safety requirements. It takes great courage for them to step aside and enter into the mystery of these ancient skills.

Often, as they relax and trust, they cry, releasing years of grief. Many of them have lived with broken hearts and souls for half a lifetime and kept a brave lid on their feelings. When we share as a group, it is powerful and humbling.

The Soul Midwives' School offers professional training and mentoring programmes for Soul Midwives. Students are mainly from the UK, but they also come from as far away as the USA, Canada, South Africa, New Zealand and Europe. The training is recognized by many hospices and mainstream organizations in the UK and abroad.

The school also goes on tour and takes training to hospices, care homes and hospitals throughout the UK.

People from all walks of life and of all ages are welcomed on our introductory days. From these, a significant number become practising Soul Midwives.

Through our links with practitioners in other branches of medicine, we are constantly developing and expanding our course material.

We are deeply committed to the service we offer and take a very practical and heart-based approach to the spiritual and sensitive aspects of death and dying.

Courses

Introduction to Soul Midwifery

This is a one-day introduction workshop covering the role and scope of Soul Midwifery. It is an exciting, hands-on, experiential day exploring the dying process and Soul Midwifery concepts and techniques to assist the dying.

Practitioner Course: Level 1

This three-day course is designed to give you the basic skills you will need in order to become a Soul Midwife.

Many students on this course are already working as carers, therapists, nurses, doctors or priests and celebrants and are seeking to extend their existing skills. However, anyone who feels called to do this work will be accepted without prior experience, as long as their motives for the work are compassion, integrity and devotion.

This is a certificated course leading to registration and eligibility for insurance (at the discretion of the insurance company) and membership of the Soul Midwives' forum for support, mentoring and continued professional development courses and study days.

After this course we recommend that you are an apprentice Soul Midwife until you have worked (and documented) supporting six friends until their deaths.

Practitioner Course: Level 2

A two-day course exploring the dynamics of the soul, the spiritual aspects of the dying process and the dynamics between the dying and the living.

International Distance Practitioner Training Program

This very popular online course enables people from all over the world to study Soul Midwifery. It consists of an introductory stand-alone module and a ten-module practitioner programme.

Soul Midwife TLC Carers' Course (Gentle Dying)

The Soul Midwife TLC Carers' Course is for hospital and hospice volunteers whose role is simply to sit at the bedside providing company for those at the end of life without involving advanced Soul Midwifery skills.

Study Days

The school also offers day courses covering specific aspects of Soul Midwifery.

Distance-Learning Course

There is a full distance-learning course for Soul Midwives throughout the world and a growing number of Soul Midwife ambassadors who are able to offer local advice and support.

Australia
Ann Rayner: ann.rayner@y7mail.com

Canada
Louise O'Brien: bluecottage@shaw.ca

New Zealand
Sorrel Renton Green (Dove House, Eastern Bays Hospice, Auckland): sorrelrentongreen@mac.com

Northern Cyprus
Helen Fields: www.letstalkaboutdeath.co.uk

South Africa

Cameron Hogg (spiritual director of hospiceWits Johannesburg):
cameronhogg@hospicewits.co.za

The United States of America

Bridget Betzer: www.anamcara.com
Virginia Farney: ginny.farney@gmail.com

CODE OF CONDUCT FOR THE SOUL MIDWIVES' SCHOOL

- I will respect the confidentiality and dignity of my 'friends' and their loved ones at all times.

- I will work harmoniously with all associated health professionals, doctors and nurses and the friends' carers in all settings and facilities.

- I will refrain from sharing my own religious beliefs and will follow the Soul Midwives' Foundation's non-denominational approach.

- I will respect my friend's faith as part of the Soul Midwives' Foundation's acceptance of all faiths.

- I will be supportive of other Soul Midwives within the Foundation.

- I will refrain from diagnosing illness or claiming to cure or heal medical conditions.

- I will not do anything that might bring Soul Midwives and their work into disrepute.

- I will only carry out treatments and give advice within an area in which I am professionally qualified.

- I will keep full and accurate records of all friends and all treatments carried out and store records in accordance with the Data Protection Act 1998 [or relevant legislation].

- I will obtain the requisite insurance to cover my Soul Midwifery practice.

- Having completed the Practitioner training, if I have not previously worked with the dying in a hospice/care home environment, I will complete a period of apprenticeship by completing six case studies with friends and having them accepted by the Soul Midwives' School as being of an appropriate standard, and I will volunteer to work with the dying in a local hospice/care home for a minimum of six months to gain experience.

- I will not teach Soul Midwifery until I have completed my apprenticeship, gained my full qualification and successfully completed a Soul Midwives' teaching course.

- I will not infringe upon the intellectual property of the Soul Midwives' School and will not use any copyrighted materials from the Soul Midwives' School curriculum, nor will I teach Soul Midwives' School copyrighted materials to other people until I have successfully completed a Soul Midwives' teaching course or have first obtained written permission from the Soul Midwives' School.

❧ INDEX ❧

clove oil 208
coffee tincture 193
colour therapy 122–3
comforting 23
  tools 201, 203
  with touch *see* hand holding;
    massage; touch
Coming Forth by Day (Egyptian *Book of
  the Dead*) 6–7, 8, 241
compassion 18, 29, 30, 33, 38, 48, 137,
  145, 169–70, 205
  fatigue 209
  see also love
consciousness
  death as a transition in xi, 10–11
  expansion of 82
  heart as centre of 5
  loss of 147
  mystery of 5
  singing bowls as tools of 83
  subtle 11
  survival of xx, 10
Constantine, Emperor 4
conversation with the dying 156–8
crab apple flower remedy 194
Curanderismo 13–14, 211

D
Dade, Dee 70–71
dark night of the soul 147–8, 213
death
  acceptance of mortality 69–70
  accidental 55
  art of dying 4
  cultural and religious beliefs 174–6
  documentation 185, 238
  dying to the old 227–8
  and evolution 227–8
  exercise in leaving life behind 56–7
  exercise in looking back before 57
  experiences at the very end 59–60
  and fear 55
  and the four elements *see* elements,
    four
  giving permission to die 162–4, 174
  how it feels emotionally 55–6

  as an illusion xx
  journey of *see* journey of death
  legal requirements 185, 238
  medical indicators of 178
  mysteries of the dying hour 20, 54
  and the point of surrender 55
  preparing for *see* preparation work
    for death
  process *see* dying process
  requirements of different faiths
    238–9
  and the separation of spirit and soul
    60–61, 181
  signs that death is near 146–50
  suicide 99
  and transcendence 55
  as a transition in consciousness xi,
    10–11
  and vibration shifts 58–9
  and visits from beyond the threshold
    186
  working with the dying *see* care of
    the dying
death-rattle 173
defecation 150
dream diaries 73
dreams
  with Air withdrawal 105
  dream state healing work 85
  with Earth withdrawal 101
  entering a dying person's dream
    state at the threshold 173
  with Fire withdrawal 104
  with Water withdrawal 103
drowsiness 147
dying process xx–xxi, 54–5, 99–141
  active dying phase 24–7, 86, 146–50
  entering and crossing the threshold
    167–8, 171–80 *see also* sacred
    threshold
  leaving of soul/spirit energy from the
    body 176–7
  opening of the chakras 106–11
  pre-active dying stage 22–4
  separation of spirit and soul 60–61,
    181

❧ NOTES ❧

NOTES

NOTES

❧ NOTES ❧

NOTES

ABOUT THE AUTHOR

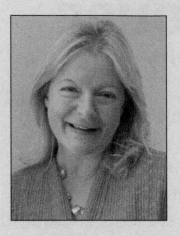

Felicity Warner comes from a long tradition of original thinkers dedicated to keeping perennial wisdom alive in contemporary thinking.

For more than 30 years, her study of philosophy, spirituality and complementary medicine has been inspired by Plato, Asclepius, Jung and the mystery traditions of both East and West.

Felicity runs the Soul Midwives School in Dorset, UK, and lectures in hospitals, hospices, universities and in the community.

Her current research involves working with aromatic plant oils and their effects on the human energy field, which she combines with her healing and soul ministry.